second edition

the
anatomy
colouring
and
workbook

For Elsevier:

Associate Editor: Siobhan Campbell
Development Editor: Veronika Watkins
Project Manager: Gail Wright
Senior Designer: Sarah Russell
Illustration Managers: Gillian Richards and Kirsteen Wright

second edition

the anatomy colouring and workbook

Stuart Porter BSc(Hons) GradDipPhys MCSP SRP CertMHS

Lecturer in Physiotherapy, School of Health Care Professions,
University of Salford, UK

Cartoons
David Banks

Illustrations
Samantha Elmhurst

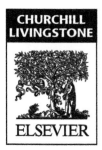

CHURCHILL LIVINGSTONE

ELSEVIER

EDINBURGH LONDON NEW YORK OXFORD PHILADELPHIA ST LOUIS SYDNEY TORONTO 2008

CHURCHILL
LIVINGSTONE
ELSEVIER

© 2008, Elsevier Limited. All rights reserved.

No part of this publication may be reproduced, stored in a retrieval system, or transmitted in any form or by any means, electronic, mechanical, photocopying, recording or otherwise, without the prior permission of the Publishers. Permissions may be sought directly from Elsevier's Health Sciences Rights Department, 1600 John F. Kennedy Boulevard, Suite 1800, Philadelphia, PA 19103-2899, USA: phone: (+1) 215 239 3804; fax: (+1) 215 239 3805; or, e-mail: *healthpermissions@elsevier.com*. You may also complete your request on-line via the Elsevier homepage (http://www.elsevier.com), by selecting 'Support and contact' and then 'Copyright and Permission'.

First edition 2002
Second edition 2008

ISBN 978-0-7506-7541-3

British Library Cataloguing in Publication Data
A catalogue record for this book is available from the British Library

Library of Congress Cataloging in Publication Data
A catalog record for this book is available from the Library of Congress

Notice
Neither the Publisher nor the Author assumes any responsibility for any loss or injury and/or damage to persons or property arising out of or related to any use of the material contained in this book. It is the responsibility of the treating practitioner, relying on independent expertise and knowledge of the patient, to determine the best treatment and method of application for the patient.

The Publisher

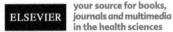
The Publisher's policy is to use paper manufactured from sustainable forests

Contents

About the author

Stuart Porter graduated from Manchester Royal Infirmary School of Physiotherapy in 1987 and later obtained a BSc(Hons) degree in Health Studies from Salford University. He went to work at Wrightington Hospital near Wigan, specialising in rheumatology and orthopaedics, later working at Ormskirk District General Hospital in Lancashire as a Senior 1 in Orthopaedics. He has lectured since 1997 in physiotherapy at the University of Salford. For 3 years he was the physiotherapist to the England women's football team. He is currently studying for a PhD in exercise compliance in ankylosing spondylitis. He now lives in Lancashire with his wife and three daughters.

Note for the second edition

It was always my intention to create a book that was fun and made anatomy memorable. Now that *The Anatomy Colouring and Workbook* is in its second edition, I have been able to expand it and add sections on the brain and respiratory system as well as a photographic atlas, which adds an extra dimension to the textbook.

I am gratified that the book is now in its second edition and I hope it continues to help students of anatomy wherever they may be.

These are the changes that I have made for this edition:

1. two new chapters on the brain and respiratory system
2. more answers are now included
3. quick-reference muscle tables are included throughout the book
4. high-resolution bony and surface anatomy photographs are included.

Acknowledgements

We rarely pause to thank the people that matter. This is the best chance I will get, so I will take a little of your time to recognise the people that have made a difference in my life, and to whom I owe it all.

To Heidi, Siobhan and Veronika at Elsevier.

To my parents, Brian and Winifred, for believing in me; to my late mother-in-law, Jessica, whom I miss terribly; to my sister, Lynn; to Mark, for 35 years of friendship. To my students past and future, from whom I learn so much.

To my wife and daughters – sanity in a world gone crazy.

Introduction

OK, so you want to learn anatomy …

Maybe you need to learn it as part of your degree course, maybe you are about to commence university and just want a head start. Maybe you need a quick revision guide as those exams get ever closer. In any event this book should act as a useful study guide.

It contains plenty of pictures and rhymes which students have found useful in the past to help you get to grip with the important aspects of this fascinating but tricky subject.

THE DESIGN OF THE ANATOMY WORKBOOK

The chapters follow this formula

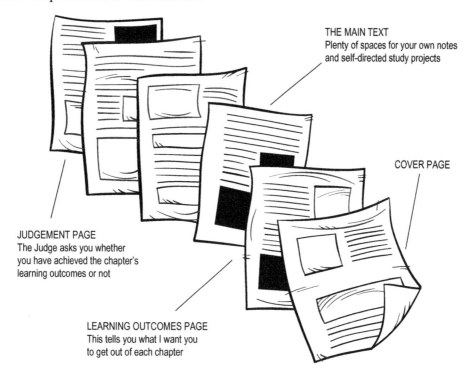

THE MAIN TEXT
Plenty of spaces for your own notes and self-directed study projects

COVER PAGE

JUDGEMENT PAGE
The Judge asks you whether you have achieved the chapter's learning outcomes or not

LEARNING OUTCOMES PAGE
This tells you what I want you to get out of each chapter

In the workbook I use friendly language, jokes and rhymes. This makes your learning easier and more fun. Remember though that you must not write in this style at exam time or in an assignment.

Answers to the self-directed study projects appear after the relevant project in the book.

This workbook should give you a clear study guide about the important points in anatomy. Study and revision needs a structure if it is to be productive – now you have a framework to build your revision upon. After several months as a student, my files were a total mess; this is my attempt to put information together in an organised way to make life as smooth as possible for you. I hope that the workbook makes your academic life a little easier.

People in the workbook to help you study

These symbols identify special tasks, tips or projects throughout the workbook.

Each chapter starts with **learning outcomes**.

The projects that you will need to complete as **self-directed study** are highlighted by this symbol.

The stressed-out student appears from time to time to help you remember the silly rhymes and word games that you will find useful.

The judge appears at the end of each chapter to assess whether you have achieved the learning outcomes that were set.

Professor. This guy appears every now and again to offer you some wise information.

This indicates where you can **colour in the illustrations** yourself to help you learn more easily.

Learning outcomes

After studying this chapter you should be able to:

1. Describe the anatomical position.

2. Describe the terms such as medial, lateral, proximal, distal and so on, included in this chapter.

3. Be able to describe the planes of the body.

4. Be able to describe the movements listed in this chapter, e.g. flexion, abduction, etc.

5. Be able to classify the types of synovial joint.

6. Be able to classify types of bones.

7. Know the functions of the skeleton.

8. Be able to describe the features of bones listed.

9. Be able to classify morphology of muscle.

10. Be able to describe the function and components of a synovial joint.

Finding your way in anatomy

As with any long journey, you need to know your starting point. Anatomy has its own language and terminology, which is really not difficult once you understand the basics; that's what the next few pages are all about. Even before this, though, you need to understand an important concept.

Experiment …

Put your hand on a table palm downwards .... point to the top of your hand

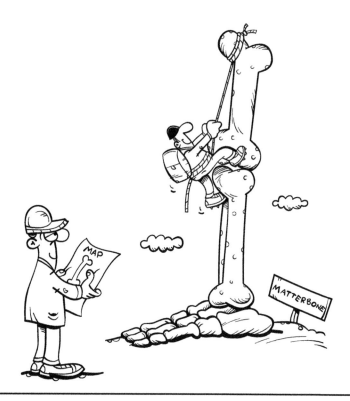

Now place your hand palm up .... point to the top of your hand

Do you see the problem?

It is difficult to know which surface to call the top and which to call the bottom of the hand. A similar mix-up in a patient lying on an operating table could have disastrous consequences. Therefore, in anatomy and medicine, all descriptions assume the ANATOMICAL POSITION; this is shown below.

THE ANATOMICAL POSITION

Person stands erect; facing forwards feet point forwards slightly apart, arms hanging down by the sides with palms facing forwards.

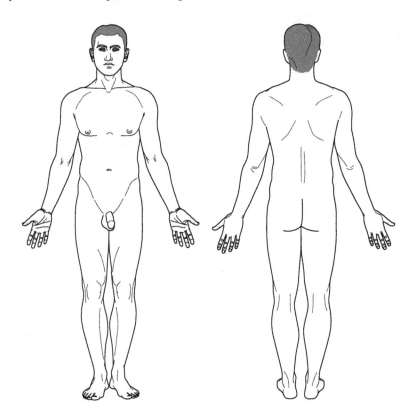

Is all our anatomy the same?

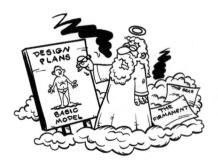

Thankfully, we are all individuals with different appearances and characteristics. Being different gives each of us a unique identity of which we are proud. Yet, at the same time, we all have the same anatomical design plans. You may find it strange to learn that there are anatomical differences from person to person. Some people have extra bones (not major ones). Some people have muscles that are absent in others, and a nerve that supplies a particular muscle in

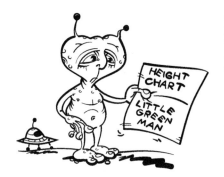

your arm may not be exactly the same as the same nerve in your friend's arm. All of these minor variations may be considered normal. However, we are basically put together in the same way, and the study of anatomy is possible, unless of course you end up working in outer space treating space aliens – I can't help you there!

Little green men may not have the same anatomy as you and me.

Directions in anatomy

Now we have a map (anatomical position), we need some directions.

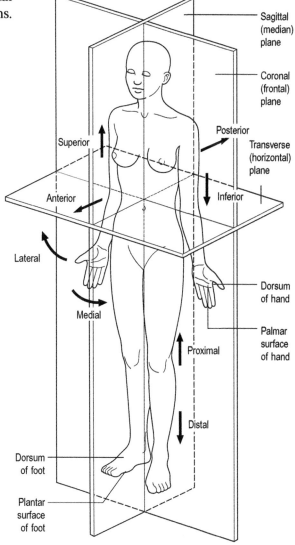

☞ Remember a piece of fluff in close proximity to your belly button (**umbilicus**).

☞ Remember painting your **fingernails a dist**urbing (distal) colour.

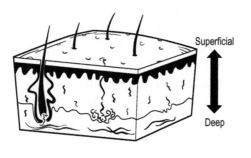

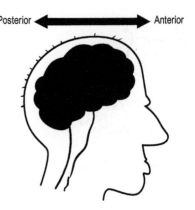

Find definitions for the following terms and put them into your own words.

Inferior   Superior

Anterior   Posterior

Medial   Lateral

Prone   Supine

Deep   Superficial

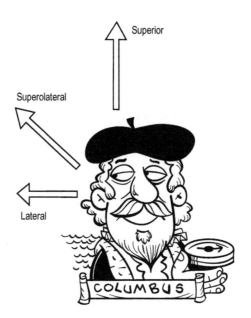

Combinations of words are sometimes used to describe positions, rather like points on a compass. So a cross between north and west is northwest, a cross between superior and lateral is superolateral. So, for example, your ear is superolateral to your mouth.

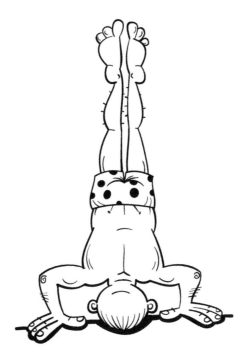

Important – no matter what position you put yourself in, all measurements in anatomy are taken from the anatomical position.

Test yourself

Place an X:
  Superior to letter A
  Distal to letter B
  Lateral to letter C
  Proximal to letter D
  Inferior to letter E
  Inferomedial to letter A.

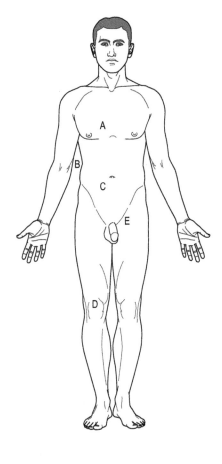

The planes of the body

If we take a human body we can cut it in various directions.

Using anatomical terminology, describe these three sections of the head

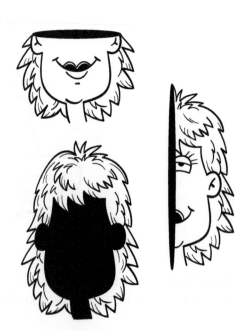

Professor's tip

Remember Sagittarius the Archer firing an arrow directly at you, the arrow would pass through you in a sagittal plane.

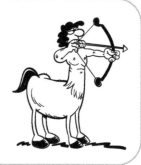

Important point: in anatomy 'the leg' refers to the knee downwards, including the foot. The part between the hip and the knee is called the thigh.

This does not really matter when you are speaking to your patients but in examinations and assignments you should use the correct terminology.

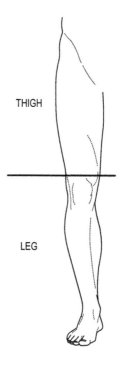

THIGH

LEG

Meet Jenny

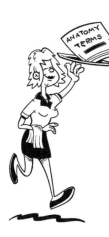

Jenny is a waitress. Try this fill in the blanks test to see if you understand anatomical terminology.

☞ Jenny wakes up in the morning. She is lying on her back, in a ①............... position.

☞ She sits up and looks at her watch. She notices that her fingernails need cutting. Her fingernails are ②........... to her wrists.

☞ She goes into the bathroom and cleans her teeth. She notices a pain in her shoulder, which is ③................. to her elbow.

☞ She looks in the mirror and wishes she had not been partying last night, she has bags under or ④............. to her eyes.

☞ She plucks her eyebrows which are ⑤............. to her eyes.

☞ She goes to work and her first job is to lift a tray of drinks above her head. In this position her hand is ⑥............... to her elbow and ⑦............... to her shoulder.

☞ She then puts her arm down to her side. In this position her hand is ⑧............... to her elbow and ⑨.............. to her shoulder.

☞ As she is serving, she bangs her thigh on the table. Later she notices a bruise on the outside of her thigh, or on the ⑩.............. aspect.

Answers

① supine. ② distal or inferior. ③ proximal or superior. ④ inferior. ⑤ superior. ⑥ inferior or distal. ⑦ inferior or distal. ⑧ same as ⑥. ⑨ same as ⑦. ⑩ lateral. ⑦ and ⑧ were trick questions, the position of her hand is irrelevant, her hand will always be distal to her shoulder no matter what she does with it!

MOVEMENTS IN ANATOMY

Movements in an antero-posterior direction (i.e. median or paramedian plane)

(Do not forget that all movements are in relation to the anatomical position.)

☞ **Flexion** The bending of two body segments so that their two anterior or posterior surfaces are brought together.

☞ **Extension** Movement in the opposite direction to flexion.

☞ **Plantarflexion** For the ankle, this refers to pointing the foot downwards (when wearing stilettos your foot is plantarflexed). Pulling the foot towards the body is dorsiflexion.

Movements in a lateral direction (i.e. in a coronal plane)

☞ **Abduction** Movement of a body segment away from the mid-line.

☞ **Adduction** Movement opposite to abduction.

☞ **Lateral flexion** The term used to describe sideways bending of the trunk to the left or the right.

☞ **Circumduction** A combination of all movements, e.g. the shoulder circumducts when you swim the crawl (it moves in a cone). This is commonest at the hip and shoulder joints.

Rotation

Movement of a bone around a central axis without displacement of that axis is rotation, it may be inward (medial/internal) or outward (lateral/external).

☞ **Supination** This describes the act of turning the palm towards the ceiling when standing (it is also occasionally used to describe movements in the foot).

☞ **Pronation** The opposite of supination, where the palm is turned down towards the floor.

Special movements

Some movements do not fall into any of the above categories.

☞ **Elevation** Raising a part, e.g. shrugging your shoulders is elevation of the shoulder girdle.

☞ **Depression** The opposite to elevation.

☞ **Protraction** Moving a part forwards, e.g. rounding your shoulders.

☞ **Retraction** The opposite to protraction.

☞ **Inversion** Turning the sole of your foot inwards as if looking at your sole is inversion.

☞ **Eversion** The opposite to inversion.

The main types of synovial joint

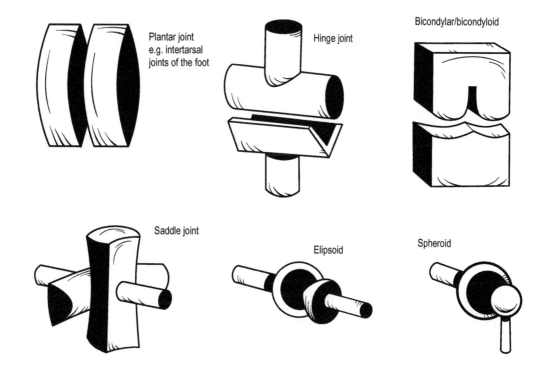

Plantar joint
e.g. intertarsal
joints of the foot

Hinge joint

Bicondylar/bicondyloid

Saddle joint

Elipsoid

Spheroid

CLASSIFICATION OF BONES

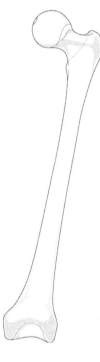

Long bones, e.g. femur or humerus (longer than they are wide).

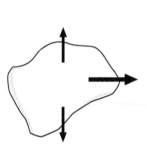

Short bones, e.g. cuboid in the foot (do not have a long axis).

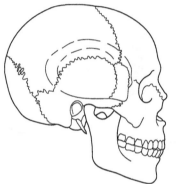

Flat bones, e.g. bones of the skull.

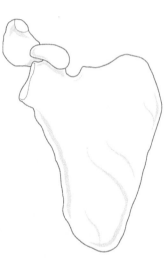

Irregular bones, e.g. scapula (shoulder blade) and pelvis (don't fit any category).

Professor asks

1. Look in a butcher's shop window – what colour is a fresh bone?
2. When you start looking at skeletons in the classroom, you will notice that they are chalky and white. Why?
3. Why is a broken bone painful?

Answers
1. Living bone is pink.
2. Classroom skeletons have lost their organic parts; all that remains are hard mineral salts.
3. Bone is alive, highly vascular and surrounded by a sensitive membrane – the periosteum.

THE TASKS OF THE SKELETON

Millions of years ago, humans opted for an internal or endoskeleton. This has good and bad points, but at least we don't have to shed our skeleton whenever we wish to grow, like insects do.

Our skeleton has many functions:

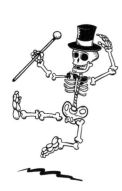

1. Support – the framework of the body, most muscles attach to bones
2. Movement – bones end in joints, so the shape of the bones often dictates how we can move
3. Protection – vital organs such as the brain are encased in bone, lungs are encased by ribs, and the uterus in the female is protected by the bowl of the pelvis
4. Mineral reservoirs of calcium, phosphorus, sodium, potassium and so on, are stored in bone. They can be moved around and mobilised when necessary, e.g. calcium is removed from the bones of the pregnant mother to give to the foetus. This is an important point since osteoporosis is an increasingly common condition. This is where the bone begins to lose mineral density either through lack of weight-bearing exercise (e.g. a patient on bed rest, or in a wheelchair) or through hormonal changes
5. Haemopoiesis (red marrow produces red blood cells).

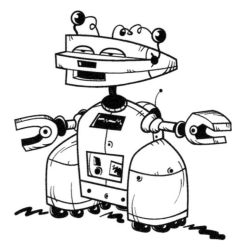

An external (exoskeleton) would look good but you would need to shed it in order to grow – ask any insect what a pain that is!

Table 0.1 Features of the bones

Projections	For articulation (connection) with other bones
	Head, condyle, facet
	For ligament/muscle attachment
	Trochanter, Tuberosity,
	Epicondyle, Tubercle
Elongated projection	Process
	Spine
	Ramus
Ridges	Crest, Line, Ridge, Spine
Depression	Facet
	Smooth, slight depression
	Fossa
	Depression
	Fovea
	Pit for ligament attachment
	Sulcus
	Groove or channel
Holes	Foramen = hole
	Meatus = canal

Test yourself …

1. Why do bones have these lumps and bumps?
2. How can an archaeologist tell by looking at a femur whether the person was a muscular individual?
3. Why do you need to know where they are?

Answers

1. Bones possess lumps and bumps in response to attachment of ligaments, muscles or tendons. Basically if a bone possesses a bump – something attaches to it!
2. An archaeologist or forensic scientist can estimate how muscular an individual was by examining the size and development of bony prominences; bodybuilders, for example, will have larger bumps than physically inactive people such as university lecturers!
3. You need to know what is normal before you can hope to identify the abnormal.

COMPONENTS OF A MUSCLE

Connective tissue coverings (fascia)

Each skeletal muscle is composed of many separate fibres; these are bound together by sheets of connective tissue called fascia. The fascia that encases an entire muscle is called the epimysium. Fascia also penetrates muscle, separating muscle fibres into bundles called fasciculi.

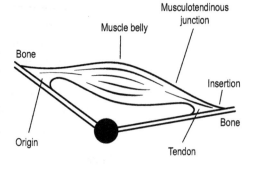

Muscle attachments

Muscles are anchored to the skeleton by extensions of the layers of fascia enveloping and within them. These extensions may attach directly to the periosteum (bone lining) or they may blend into a strong fibrous connection (tendons). Tendons may be quite short or may be up to 30 cm long; tendons that take the shape of broad sheets are called aponeuroses.

MORPHOLOGY (SHAPES) OF MUSCLES

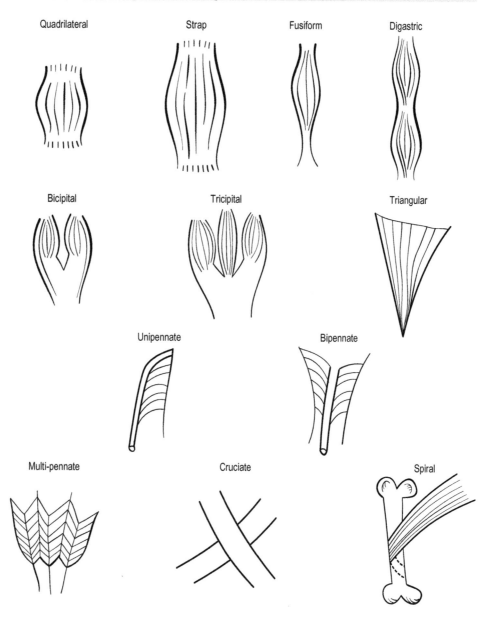

Quadrilateral

Strap

Fusiform

Digastric

Bicipital

Tricipital

Triangular

Unipennate

Bipennate

Multi-pennate

Cruciate

Spiral

Think about it

When a muscle contracts, it shortens in length and pulls its ends closer together. If the muscle is attached to either end of two bones, it pulls their ends closer together.

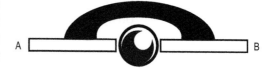

A

B

Below, I want you to draw how bones A and B would look when muscle C contracts …

1. If bone A is immobile

2. If bone B is immobile

3. If both bones are immobile.

Answers
If bone A is immobile, bone B will move in an arc around the central joint.

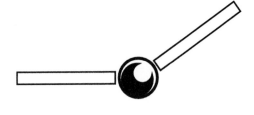

If bone B is immobile, bone A will move in an arc around the central joint.

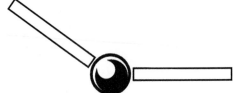

If both bones are immobile, then the net result will be compression at the joint. Muscles often work simultaneously across joints to give them stability, e.g. biceps and triceps in the arm.

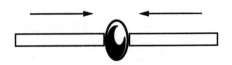

If both muscles above contract simultaneously, what will be the effect on the joint in the centre?

Answer
Joint stabilisation.

A. – If this muscle contracts, what will it do to joints 1 and 2? Draw the result below.

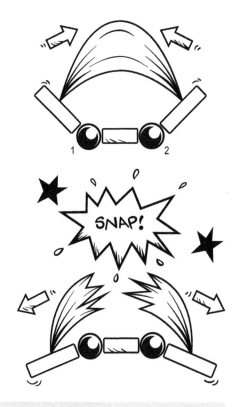

B. – Draw the position into which you would put the bones if you wished to stretch or even snap (rupture) the muscle.

TYPES OF MOVEMENT

This can take a little effort to grasp so I would like you to meet Fred. Fred is a student. I will use a 1-hour period in his life to attempt to explain various types of joint movement.

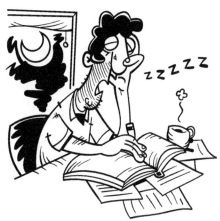

Fred was up studying until 2.00 a.m. (As all you students are!) He has an exam today.

He is so tired he fell asleep with his arm on his textbook last night.

His flatmate needs the book and so, without waking Fred, the flatmate lifts up Fred's arm and removes the book .... This is an example of a **passive movement** on Fred's part. It required no muscle action by Fred even though Fred's shoulder joint moved.

Fred begins to wake up but he is late for the exam, his friend helps to dress him and helps him to lift his arm into his pullover, Fred does some of the work and so does his friend .... This is an example of an **active assisted movement**. Fred's own muscles did some but not all of the work.

Fred is now in the bathroom and reaches up to grab the toothpaste .... This is an **active movement** – Fred's own muscles controlled the movement.

Fred now rushes down the hall and tries to open the door, it sticks and he has to push it quite hard …. This is a **resisted movement** – Fred's muscles had to work against an external force.

(Fred passed his exam.)

Please note that any similarity to any student living or dead is purely coincidental. No student would ever be so silly as to leave revision this late or oversleep for an exam …. would you … hello …?

TYPES OF MUSCLE WORK

There now follows a practical demonstration involving something very dear to my heart – food.

You will need a meat pie.

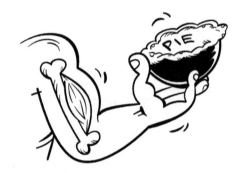

Let us look at a single muscle, in this case the biceps brachii. At rest, the muscle is relaxed and generates no tension. Lift the pie towards your mouth, the biceps contracts and flexes your elbow.

During this movement, the biceps shortens in length. This is called a *concentric* contraction. As you lower your arm back down to replace the pie (extend the elbow) it is still the same muscle doing the work but this time it is slowly paying out tension and thus lengthening. This is an *eccentric* contraction. Concentric and eccentric contractions are collectively termed isotonic contractions because there is a change in the length of the muscle.

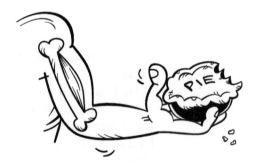

Now, let's assume that the pie has been glued to the table – a distressing concept I know. You try to pick it up and you can feel the tension and see the contraction in the biceps, but the pie does not move, and the elbow remains motionless: this is called an *isometric* contraction. The muscle has contracted but has not changed in length.

So, to summarise the types of muscle contraction.

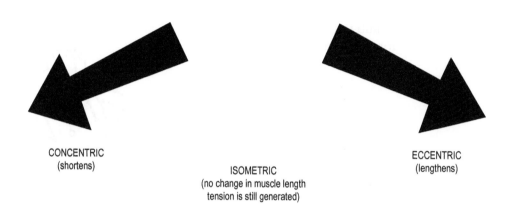

ISOTONIC
(change in muscle length)

CONCENTRIC
(shortens)

ISOMETRIC
(no change in muscle length
tension is still generated)

ECCENTRIC
(lengthens)

How can I remember what an eccentric contraction looks like?

Imagine one of your *eccentric* lecturers who is handing an assignment back to you, he slowly *lowers* the assignment on to the table suggesting that maybe you should be *paying* for extra tuition, whilst trying to control his rage – this is an *eccentric* contraction of the biceps as it slowly controls the movement and *pays* out its length.

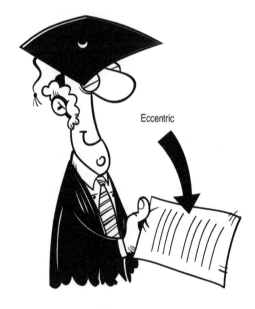

Eccentric

BURSA (PLURAL BURSAE)

There are parts of the body that move against each other constantly. Much as a car needs lubrication with oil so do these parts of the body. The answer is a bursa; here is what a bursa does …

Rub your hands together quickly for one minute.
What happens?

1. They get hot.
2. It hurts.
3. You would quickly wear away your skin!

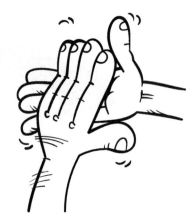

Now, put a bottle of ketchup or a can of cola between your hands and rub them as you did before, what happens?

1. The can or bottle rolls with your skin.
2. Your hands do not get hot.
3. You could keep going all day without wearing away your skin.

This is the best way I can think of to describe how a bursa works. A bursa is an expansion of synovial membrane that is found at sites of potential friction, e.g. between your Achilles tendon and your calcaneus (heel bone). Bursae are lubricated on their inner walls by synovial fluid.

By rolling between the two structures, friction is kept to a minimum and damage is prevented – think about how many thousands of times per day your tissues might rub against one another.

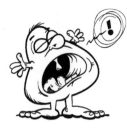

Meet Billy Bursa. As you can see, he is inflamed. This is known as bursitis. What would you have to do to him to make him irritable?

1. Stretch him   4. Infect him
2. Overuse him   5. All of the above
3. Squash him

Answer
All of the above could give Billy bursitis.

COMPONENTS OF A TYPICAL SYNOVIAL JOINT

You *must* know the function of each of these structures in a normal joint before you can understand how they are affected by various conditions and diseases.

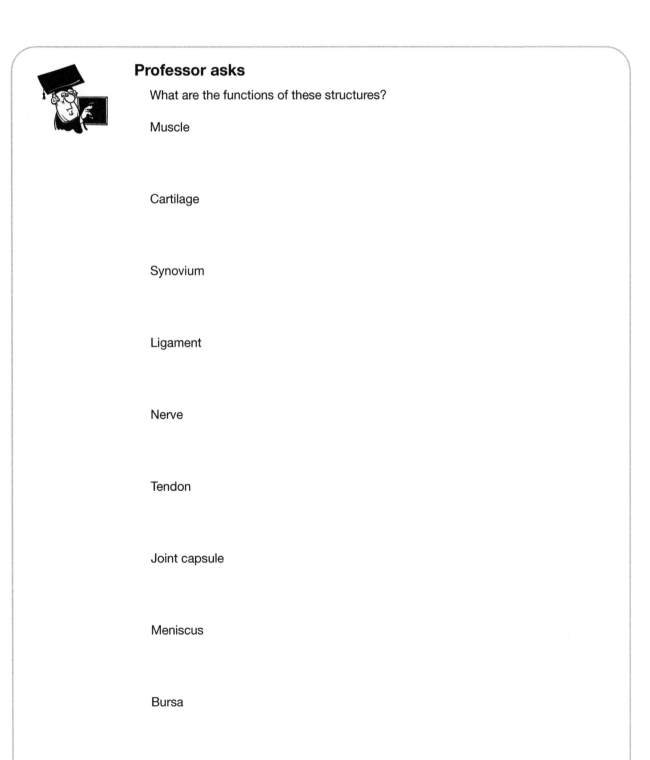

Professor asks

What are the functions of these structures?

Muscle

Cartilage

Synovium

Ligament

Nerve

Tendon

Joint capsule

Meniscus

Bursa

Judgement time

How have you done?

- ❑ It is now time for you to assess whether or not you have successfully achieved the learning outcomes that I set out at the start of this chapter.
- ❑ You need to be able to tick each box below.
- ❑ If you cannot, return to the study of the relevant section of the chapter.
- ❑ Can you describe the anatomical position?
- ❑ Can you describe the terms such as medial, lateral, proximal, distal and so on included in this chapter?
- ❑ Are you able to describe the planes of the body?
- ❑ Are you able to describe the movements listed in this chapter, e.g. flexion, abduction and so on?
- ❑ Are you able to classify the types of synovial joint found in the body?
- ❑ Are you able to classify types of bones?
- ❑ Do you know the functions of the human skeleton?
- ❑ Are you able to describe the features of bones listed?
- ❑ Are you able to classify morphology of muscle?
- ❑ Are you able to describe the function and components of a typical synovial joint?
- ❑ Can you recall the features of the bones listed?

PART **1**

Bones of the lower limb

Learning outcomes

After reading this chapter you should be able to:

1. Describe in detail the structure and function of all of the bones of the lower limb.

2. Be able to palpate these bony points

- Anterior superior iliac spine (ASIS)
- Posterior superior iliac spine (PSIS)
- Iliac crest
- Pubic tubercle
- Ischial tuberosity
- Greater trochanter
- Adductor tubercle
- Medial femoral condyle and epicondyle

- Lateral femoral condyle and epicondyle
- Medial tibial condyle
- Lateral tibial condyle
- Tibial tuberosity
- Patella
- Head of the fibula
- Medial malleolus
- Lateral malleolus
- Tuberosity of navicular
- Cuboid
- Calcaneal tuberosity
- Tubercle at base of 5th metatarsal
- Metatarsals 1–5
- Phalanges 1–5.

THE PELVIS

Anterior view

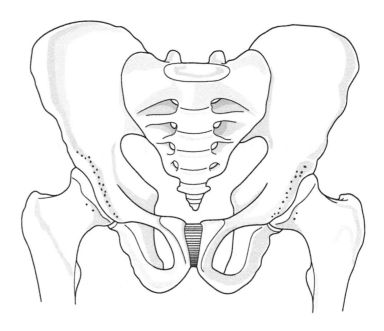

Three separate bones form the pelvis:

☞ the ilium
☞ the ischium
☞ the pubis.

The ilium is the broad, wing-like bone which features the wide, concave surfaces of the back and sides of the pelvic girdle. The ischium forms the smaller, lower portion which bears your body weight when you are sitting. The pubis creates an archway in the front of the basin which allows the urethra, blood vessels and nerves to pass through the pelvic girdle to the external genitalia and lower body. The pelvis articulates with the sacrum in the spine and to the legs through the ball-and-socket joint formed by the acetabulum of the pelvis and the head of the femur.

The pelvis – practical

1. Sit on your hands and rock from side to side. The bumps you can feel are part of the ischium called the ischial tuberosity. You have two of these and the hamstring muscles attach here.
2. Put your hands on your hips. You are now resting your hands on top of part of your ilium called the iliac crest. You have two of these. These are large wing-like bones made up of cancellous or spongy bone; these are sometimes used by surgeons to harvest bone grafts for use in other parts of the body. Anteriorly the crests end at the anterior superior iliac spines (ASIS) and posteriorly at the posterior superior iliac spines (not surprisingly known as the PSIS!).

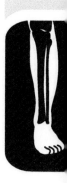

Colour in the ilium pubis and ischium in three different colours to make sure you are clear about where each one is located

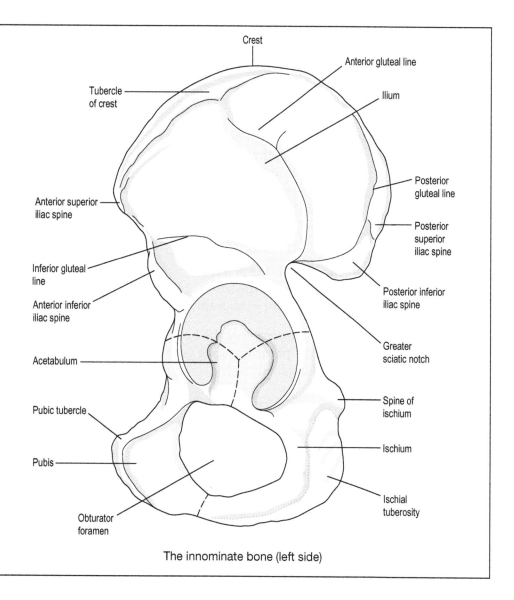

The innominate bone (left side)

Professor's tip

Think of the ilium as a box with a spine at each corner.

In a practical exam, if you are asked to locate a bony point, undress the model so that you can see and palpate (touch) the skin over the area. If you do not adequately expose the part, you may fail.

About the pelvis

The pelvis is an irregular bone. It is shaped differently in men and women, and is proportionately wider in women (sorry!). Because of this the elbow of a woman has what is known as a carrying angle, i.e. the elbow deviates away from the body to accommodate the wider pelvis. If you look at a joined pelvis, you can tell whether it came from a male or a female by looking at the angle at which the pubic bones meet in the middle: the angle is wider in a female pelvis.

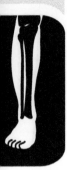

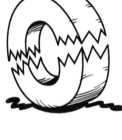

The pelvis is joined together at the front by the pubic symphysis and at the back by the sacroiliac joints. These joints do not move much, except during pregnancy and childbirth. In pregnancy, a hormone called relaxin is secreted, which makes a woman's ligaments more lax, allowing the baby to pass more easily through the pelvic girdle. This may be one of the reasons why back pain is more common during pregnancy. The pelvis may be regarded as a ring. If a ring breaks it breaks in two places (imagine snapping a polo mint) – the same is true of the pelvis.

The pelvis is the point where the spine joins onto the lower limbs. Many muscles and tendons attach to the pelvis and the pelvis is important for control of posture and balance. Trauma or osteoporosis may cause fractures (= breaks) around the pelvis. Another function of the pelvis is protection of the abdominal organs, and the socket of the hip joint (the acetabulum) is in the pelvis.

Think of the pelvis as a soup ladle containing spaghetti:

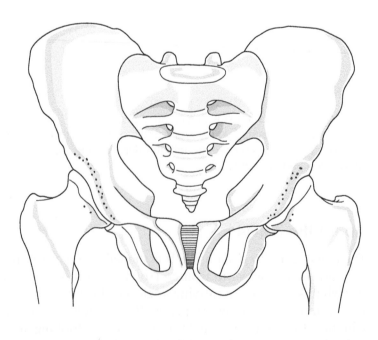

☞ the bowl = the pelvis
☞ the handle = the spine
☞ the spaghetti = abdominal contents.

In the same way that the bowl protects the spaghetti, the pelvis protects the viscera. Severe pelvic fractures may therefore have associated damage to the viscera (internal organs).

Add these labels to this diagram of a pelvis:

pubis	superior pubic ramus	posterior inferior iliac spine (PIIS)
ilium	inferior pubic ramus	posterior superior iliac spine (PSIS)
ischium	acetabulum	iliac crest
pubic symphysis	anterior inferior iliac spine (AIIS)	obturator foramen
pubic tubercle	anterior superior iliac spine (ASIS)	

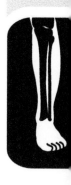

Don't panic!
Later in this book there are some actual photographs of bones and limbs with answers included for you to check your knowledge.

The sacrum

The sacrum is a wedge-shaped bone which joins the pelvis via two joints on either side (the sacroiliac joints). This is a synovial joint but it is unlike most others in that it consists of interlocking teeth with little or no movement occurring at the joint (although there is some disagreement about this fact). The sacrum is the portion of the vertebral column between the lumbar vertebrae and the structures of the coccyx. It is made up of five vertebrae which are fused together. Four pairs of holes called sacral foramina pierce the sacrum, flanking the centre.

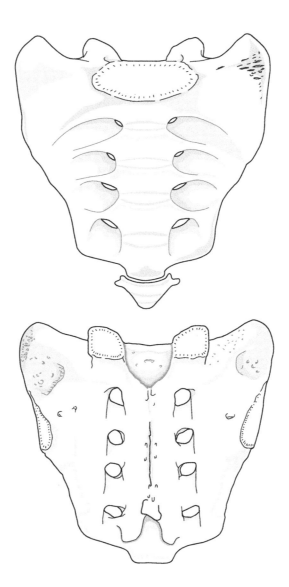

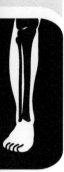

The sacrum is so-called because when they used to burn witches at the stake it was always the last bone to burn, hence it was thought sacred.

I guarantee that in times of stress, when your brain lets you down (i.e. in an exam) you will remember useless facts like these!

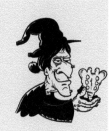

The coccyx

The coccyx is the remains of our tail from when we emerged from the seas millions of years ago. It is inferior to the sacrum. It is not really of importance except when playing Scrabble, or when it is fractured or bruised as after a fall onto the bottom, which is extremely painful. It is composed of three to five rudimentary vertebrae. Often, the first of these coccygeal vertebrae is separate, while the remainder are fused together. The articulation between the coccygeal vertebrae and the sacrum allows some flexibility in the coccyx.

In different colours on this lateral view of a pelvis, colour the

ilium
ischium
pubis

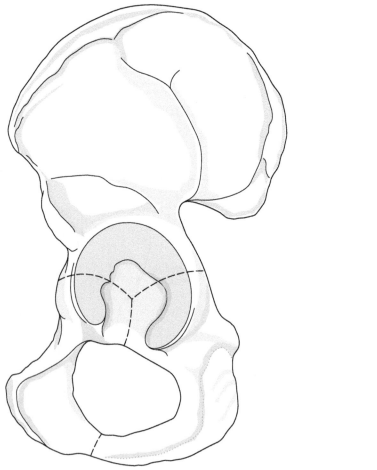

Now repeat the exercise on this anterior view.

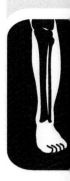

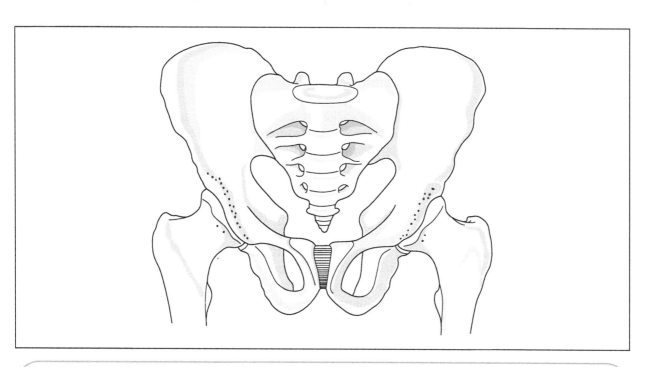

Professor's tip

Practise palpation on different bodies. We are all different and you need the experience.

Give a detailed description of the bony structure of the pelvis

Prompts
☞ Where is it?
☞ What type of bone is it?
☞ What are its major features?
☞ Which parts of the pelvis can be palpated?

Answer tips
☞ When answering this type of question, form a battle plan.
☞ What are the key features of the bone and why is each feature there?
☞ Remember, everything is there for a reason in anatomy – if something is big it's probably because something big is attached to it.
☞ What is the examiner looking for?
☞ This question is purely descriptive – so do not write essays on fractures of the pelvis, or the muscles or joints of the pelvis.
☞ Show your answer to a non-medical person – does it make sense to them?
☞ Do not use abbreviations and do not repeat yourself.
☞ Get out your highlighter pen and highlight the key words – in this case the key words are:
   Detailed – bony – pelvis.
☞ Keep re-reading the question.

THE FEMUR

The femur (thighbone) is the longest bone in the body. Superiorly it forms the hip joint, inferiorly it forms the knee joint.

The head of the femur is roughly spherical and is lined with articular cartilage; at the very top of this, a ligament (the ligamentum teres) attaches the head of the femur to the base of the socket of the hip joint (the acetabulum). The lining hyaline cartilage of the hip joint is frequently affected by degeneration (osteoarthritis). Hip replacement surgery is now very common and successful: it involves entirely replacing the head of the femur with a metal or ceramic prosthesis, and replacing the acetabulum with a tough plastic-like material.

The neck of the femur is what joins the head onto the shaft. It is important because it is one of the most common parts of the body to be affected by osteoporosis and therefore liable to fracture (break). This usually happens to elderly people, who often have other conditions and may be generally frail – it is of vital importance that these fractures are fixed surgically and the patient is 'got back on their feet' as rapidly as possible.

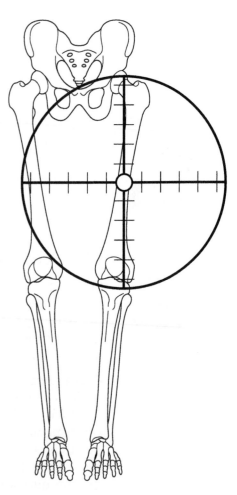

The shaft of the femur is not straight. Hold a femur and look at it sideways on, note how it is bowed; this shape is stronger than a straight tube and aids shock absorption during activities such as running. Many muscles attach themselves around the shaft of the femur, most importantly the quadriceps or thigh muscles – these extend the knee. It takes considerable force to fracture a femur unless the bone is weakened by pathology such as a tumour or osteoporosis.

The femoral condyles. A condyle is the term for a roughly rounded lump of bone, an epicondyle is the term for a lump on top of a condyle! The femur has two condyles, medial and lateral, you can feel them on your own knee. Just above the medial femoral condyle is a ridge of bone called the adductor tubercle to which attach the adductor or groin muscles. Put your hand between your knees and squeeze your thighs together: you can now see and feel your adductors working.

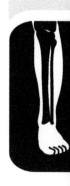

Label this femur

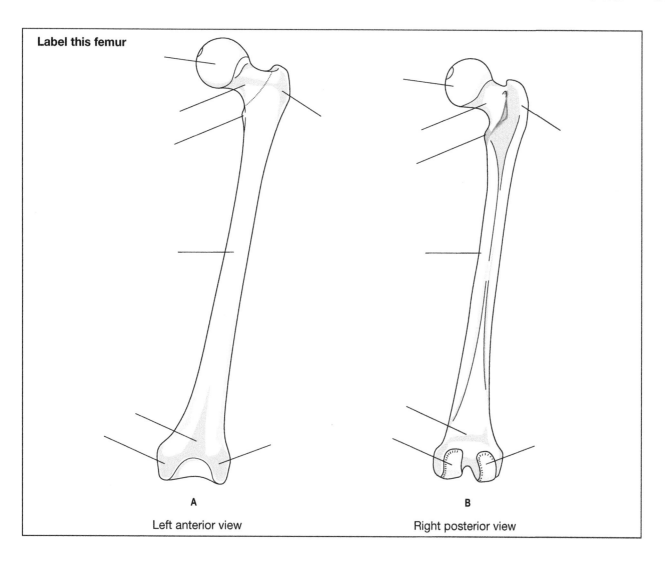

A
Left anterior view

B
Right posterior view

Professor's tip

Fractures of the femoral neck are very common indeed and you will encounter them on clinical placement. Other common osteoporotic–related fractures include vertebral body and distal radial (Colles) fractures; these all consist predominantly of cancellous bone which is most affected by osteoporosis.

How does the structure of the femur relate to its function?

Answer tips

A slightly more advanced type of question than the pelvis one – a common exam format. Do not assume that because you have read the word femur that you are safe. This question asks for more than the structure. The examiner is asking you whether you can relate form to function. This is actually quite an easy task with anatomy since all form is there for a function. So what I would suggest is that you first make a bullet point list then go into more detail for the function of each.

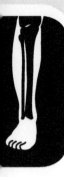

Bullet point plan
It has a spherical head → large range of movement (ROM)
It has articular cartilage → minimal friction
It has a labrum → increased stability
It has an offset femoral neck → larger ROM
It has a large greater trochanter → powerful muscle attachment
And so on.

Professor's tip

Grab a bone!

Practical sessions are a vital part of your training, but take some getting used to. Please try not to feel too embarrassed in them – you are all in the same position and you will be surprised by how quickly you get used to them.

1. Sit in a circle in your tutorial groups. Pass round a pelvis and a femur. Each person now needs to say one thing – anything – about the bone

    e.g. 'it is long'
      'it is white'
      'it has lumps on it'.

2. Anything goes. There is no such thing as a silly answer. It is *very* important that you do not feel intimidated when speaking to the rest of your group. This gets much easier with practice. Work in twos and describe the pelvis and femur to each other. Now let your partner ask you questions about the bones and how they articulate in a living body.
3. Put your hands on your own hips. What can you feel? (bony points/soft tissues).
4. Spend a few minutes comparing what you can feel compared to a classroom skeleton. Now repeat this on your colleagues.
5. Sit on your hands. What are the hard bumps that you can feel?
6. Now repeat this on your colleagues.

THE PATELLA (KNEECAP)

The patella is a small bone at the front of the knee joint which resembles an inverted teardrop. It is a sesamoid bone, connected to the joint by the medial and patellar retinaculum ligaments and to the tuberosity of the tibia by the patellar ligament (poorly named as it is actually a tendon, not a ligament).

The patella is not a shock absorber. Its function is to act as a pulley, changing the angle of pull of the patellar tendon. Without a patella, the patellar tendon would approach the tibia virtually parallel to it; this would result in an inefficient system for extending the knee. The patella is the largest sesamoid bone in the body (a bone embedded within a tendon). The posterior surface of the patella has

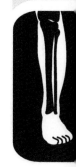

various facets which articulate with the femoral condyles throughout different parts of knee flexion/extension.

The role of the patella

A Without a patella, the tibia would just 'crash head on' into the femur when the quadriceps contracted.

B The patella alters the angle of attack of the patellar tendon, making knee extension more efficient.

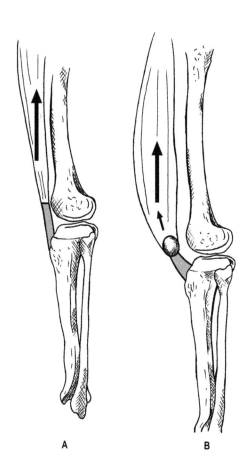

A   B

THE TIBIA AND FIBULA

You should also be able to identify the following on a tibia: intercondylar spines, lateral and medial condyles, interosseous border, soleal line, vertical line, groove for flexor hallucis longus and the fibular notch.

Superiorly the tibia forms the inferior aspect of the knee joint, and inferiorly it makes up part of the ankle (talocrural) joint. Superiorly, it fans into a broad platform which is known as the tibial plateau. On top of this is a lining of articular cartilage and two fibrocartilagenous discs called menisci (singular meniscus).

Working down the anterior border of the tibia one sees a large bump on the anterior aspect; this is called the tibial tubercle or tuberosity. This is where the patellar tendon attaches (the ligamentum patellae). You will find these types of lumps and bumps wherever powerful muscles or tough ligaments attach. These bumps are larger in men owing to their larger musculature and are even larger in bodybuilders. If you have ever had Osgood–Schlatter's disease, this is inflammation of this part of the body – common in adolescent boys. You can clearly feel your own tibial tubercle about 6 or 7 cm below the kneecap.

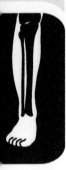

The anteromedial border is directly under the skin, which is why banging your shin hurts so much! The periosteum or membrane surrounding the bone is very sensitive to pain and has a good blood and nerve supply. (Never forget that bone is alive; a living bone is pink and vascular, not like the skeletons in the classroom, which are white and chalky – have a look in a butcher's shop at fresh bones if you don't believe me.)

Inferiorly, the tibia ends on the medial side in a rounded bone called the malleolus (plural malleoli); you can also feel this. The malleolus has a partner on the lateral aspect and together these grasp the talus, forming the ankle joint. The tibia is often fractured during sport or other accidents. Often the tibia fails to heal well because it has a poor blood supply, especially the distal portion – why do you think that is the case? Well, the answer is that the lower portion of the tibia doesn't need a good blood

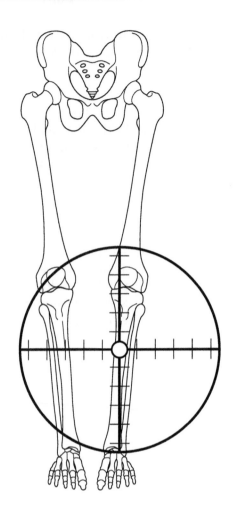

supply because by the time the muscles get down there their muscle bellies have all turned into tendons which are really pulleys that don't need a lot of blood (food). The fibula is smaller and thinner than the tibia; it joins the tibia just below the tibial plateau and is sited lateral to the tibia and its main function is to act as a site of muscle attachment. It also makes up part of the ankle joint. Like the tibia it ends in a malleolus (lateral). The head of the fibula can be felt on the lateral aspect of the leg at approximately the same level as the tibial tubercle. It is possible to move the head of the fibula with your fingers, but not a lot! The tibia and fibula are joined together by an interosseous membrane. The fibula is so named because it serves as a brace for the lower leg (fibula means 'brace').

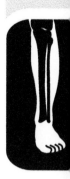

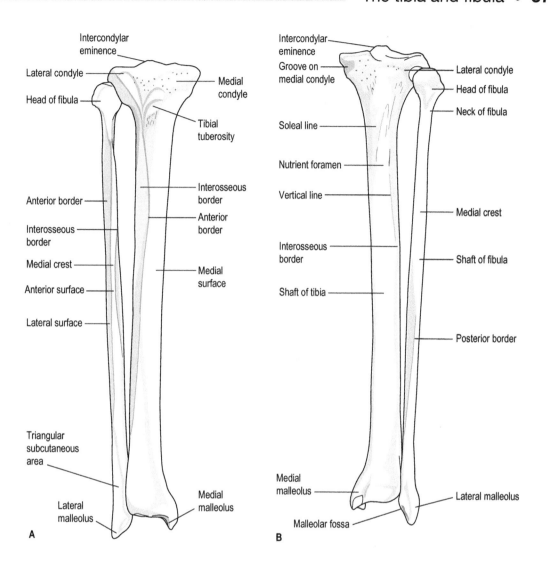

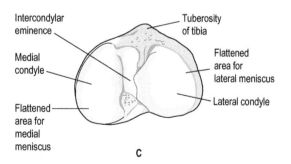

Right tibia and fibula. **A** anterior view, **B** posterior view, **C** superior view of right tibia

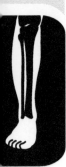

Professor's tip

Students often incorrectly palpate the lateral tibial plateau, mistaking it for the head of the fibula. Remember that the head of fibula is lower (more inferior) than you might expect, it is approximately at the same height as the tibial tubercle but at 90° to it, directly under the seam in your trousers on the lateral aspect of the leg.

Describe the tibia and fibula on a page of A4

Professor's tip

Practice makes perfect. If you will be taking a practical (viva exam) as part of your course you need to get used to talking about anatomy as well as writing about it. Use your colleagues as practice for this. You may also have the chance to do a mock exam – which will stress you out immensely but is well worthwhile – just to give you a feel for what the real thing will be like. Do not be afraid to state the obvious. At worst there is nothing lost and at best you may be right; in either case it will encourage the examiner to probe more and gets the two of you communicating – examiners are human and they do not want to fail you!

THE FOOT

Each foot is made up of 26 bones; seven of these bones form the tarsus. These tarsal bones include the navicular, the three cuneiforms, the cuboid, the talus, and the calcaneus (the heel). These tarsal bones are arranged generally in two rows, the proximal (nearer the body) and distal (nearer the toes). The distal tarsals articulate with the five metatarsals. The long metatarsals form the broad, long structure of the foot. These, in turn, articulate with the proximal phalanges (toe bones). The proximal phalanges join with the middle phalanges, which

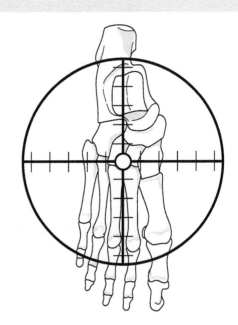

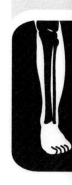

Colour each of the bones of the foot to make sure you are clear about which is which.

Right foot

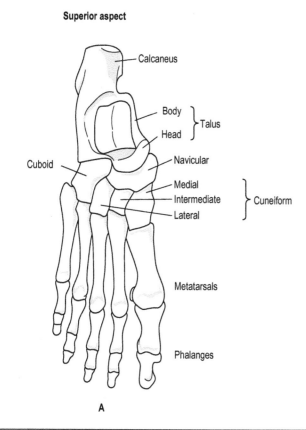

Superior aspect

Calcaneus

Body ⎱ Talus
Head ⎰

Navicular

Cuboid

Medial
Intermediate ⎱ Cuneiform
Lateral ⎰

Metatarsals

Phalanges

A

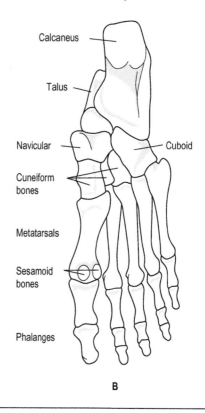

Inferior aspect

Calcaneus

Talus

Navicular

Cuboid

Cuneiform
bones

Metatarsals

Sesamoid
bones

Phalanges

B

articulate with the distal phalanges. The large toe is the exception, as it lacks a middle phalanx.

The talus

The talus from below – find the three facets for articulation with the upper surface of the calcaneus, and the articulation with the navicular bone.

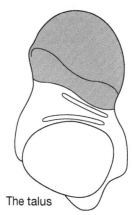

The talus

useless fact number **6,462**

Did you know that the talus is the only bone in the body which has no muscle attachments.

Try that one at the next party you go to – it will really get things going!

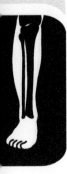

The calcaneus

Put an arrow on the diagram indicating the direction of:

The toes

The ankle joint

Find the sustentaculum tali and label it

Find the calcaneal tuberosity.

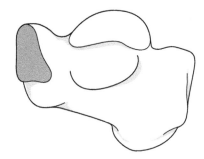

The right calcaneus

This shows the calcaneus from below (inferior view) – label it.

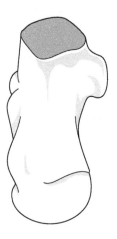

On the next pages there are diagrams of each of the tarsal bones; make your own notes on them in the spaces provided

The calcaneus

☞ Largest foot bone.
☞ Transmits weight through the heel. Articulates with talus above and cuboid in front.
☞ Often fractured by falls from a ladder onto the heels by burglars, window cleaners and peeping toms!

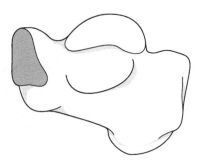

Your notes

_____

_____

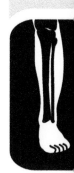

_____

_____

_____

_____

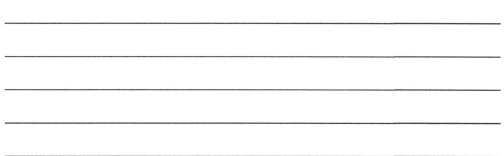

A patient who was in the navy once told me that during World War 2 the calcaneus was commonly fractured when a battleship was torpedoed – the shock being transmitted through the deck of the ship upwards through the heels – now you know.

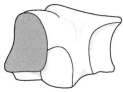

Cuboid
(Lateral view)

Your notes

_____

_____

_____

_____

_____

_____

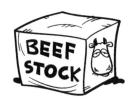

The cuboid

The cuboid looks a little like an Oxo cube

(OK maybe not.)

On the lateral side, it has a groove underneath to house the tendon of peroneus longus.

Your notes

_____

_____

_____

_____

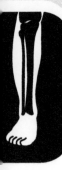

The navicular

The tuberosity of navicular can be palpated on the medial side of the foot.

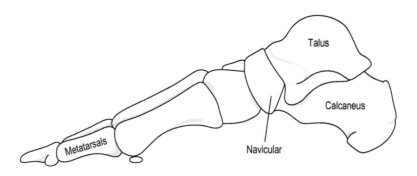

Your notes

_____

_____

_____

_____

_____

_____

The cuneiforms

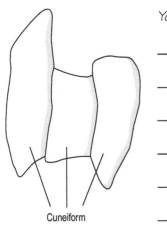

Your notes

_____

_____

_____

_____

_____

_____

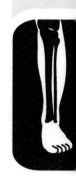

The metatarsals

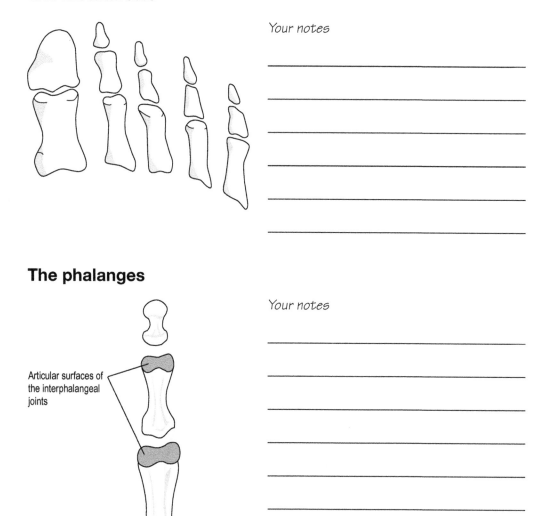

Your notes

_____

_____

_____

_____

_____

_____

The phalanges

Articular surfaces of
the interphalangeal
joints

Articular surface for
head of metatarsal

Your notes

_____

_____

_____

_____

_____

_____

_____

On a page, summarise the number, position and functions of the arches of the foot

THE ARCHES OF THE FOOT

How muscles assist in arch support

There are three main arches, a medial and lateral longitudinal and a transverse arch. They are made up from the shape of the bones and soft tissues, and muscles assist in maintaining their shape.

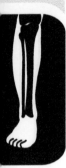

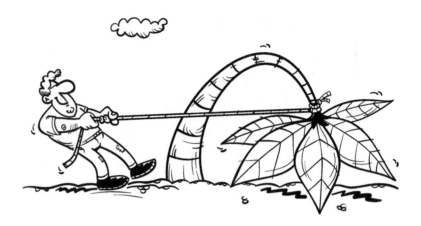

Muscles such as flexor hallucis longus.

Last time that you made an igloo you will remember that the way to get the blocks to rest securely on each other is to make them wedge shaped with the narrow part lowermost.

This is how the bones of the foot are shaped, thus helping maintain an arch shape.

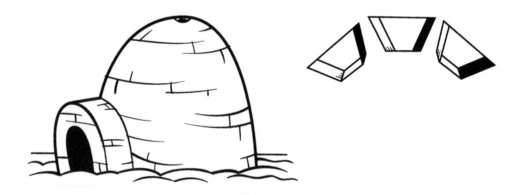

As well as the shape of the bones, ligaments and muscles act to support the arches of the foot, e.g. peroneus longus.

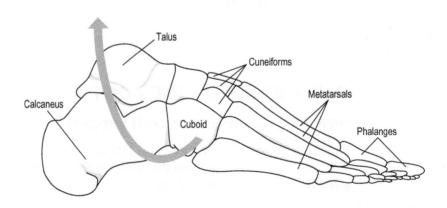

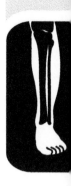

Professor's tip

Believe it or not, by the time you have been studying for a couple of months, you will know more anatomy than most patients *ever* will. Don't forget that in terms of knowledge, most patients never get past day 1 and are just as nervous and unsure as you were. So try to explain things to them in simple terms that *they* can understand – after all – that is how you remember things best isn't it?

On this leg, plot the bony points that you have learned to palpate so far

Here is a guide:

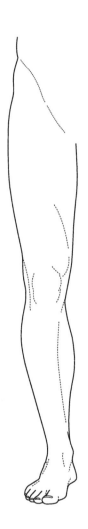

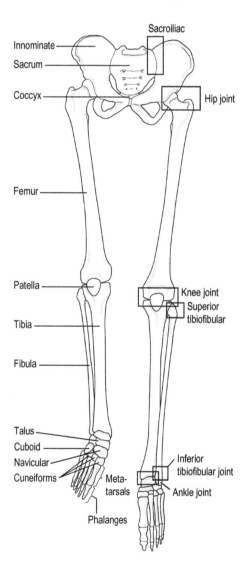

BONES   JOINTS

- Sacroiliac
- Innominate
- Sacrum
- Coccyx
- Hip joint
- Femur
- Patella
- Knee joint
- Superior tibiofibular
- Tibia
- Fibula
- Talus
- Cuboid
- Navicular
- Cuneiforms
- Meta-tarsals
- Inferior tibiofibular joint
- Ankle joint
- Phalanges

How much detail do you know?

Theory

You need to be able to describe and identify all the features of bones included in this chapter (including self-directed work).

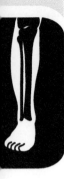

Practical – bony points and landmarks

You must be able to find these points on models of various shapes and sizes!

On three different models, find each of the bony points and get a colleague to check that you are correct

Table 1.1 On three different models, find each of the bony points and get a colleague to check that you are correct

Bony point	Model 1	Model 2	Model 3
ASIS			
PSIS			
Iliac crest			
Pubic tubercle			
Ischial tuberosity			
Greater trochanter			
Adductor tubercle			
Medial femoral condyle (plus epicondyle)			
Lateral femoral condyle (plus epicondyle)			
Medial tibial condyle			
Lateral tibial condyle			
Tibial tuberosity			
Patella			
Head of the fibula			

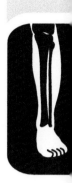

Judgement time

It is now time to see whether you have successfully achieved the learning outcomes listed at the start of this chapter. You need to be able to tick each box below before progressing further. If you cannot, go back to the relevant section of this chapter before you move on to the next chapter.

❑ Can you describe in detail the structure and function of all of the bones of the lower limb?

❑ Can you accurately palpate these bony points?

— ASIS
— PSIS
— iliac crest
— pubic tubercle
— ischial tuberosity
— greater trochanter
— adductor tubercle
— medial femoral condyle (plus epicondyle)
— lateral femoral condyle (plus epicondyle)
— medial tibial condyle
— lateral tibial condyle

— tibial tuberosity
— patella
— head of the fibula
— medial malleolus
— lateral malleolus
— tuberosity of navicular
— cuboid
— calcaneal tuberosity
— tubercle at base of 5th metatarsal
— metatarsals 1–5
— phalanges 1–5

❑ Can you identify the bony attachments/origin and insertion of the muscles and ligaments listed in the 'Joints of the lower limb' and 'Muscles of the lower limb' chapters?

2

Joints of the lower limb

Learning outcomes

After reading this chapter you should be able to:

1. Describe the structure of all joints of the lower limb including articular surfaces, movements possible, ligaments, capsule and other important features particular to that joint.

2. Describe the function of all joints of the lower limb.

3. Be able to relate 1 (above) to 2 (above).

4. Have a working knowledge of limiting factors to the movements of the joints of the lower limb.

THE HIP JOINT

The hip is a remarkable joint which possesses stability but retains mobility. It has to withstand incredible pressures during life – 18 MPa (2610 PSI) going up stairs for example. To put this in context, your car tyres typically use pressures of 200 kPa (29 PSI).

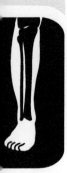

Label this diagram of a hip joint.

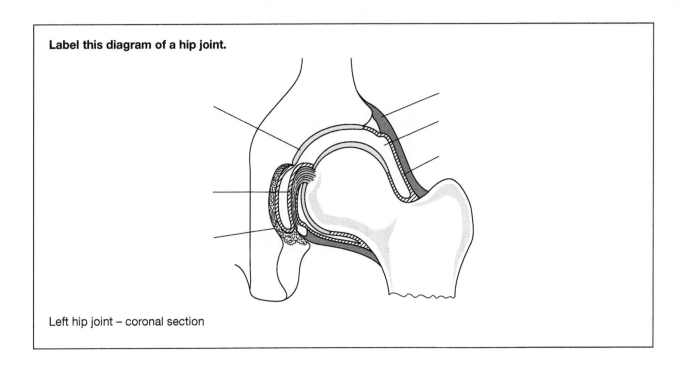

Left hip joint – coronal section

The ligaments of the hip

Label the ligaments.

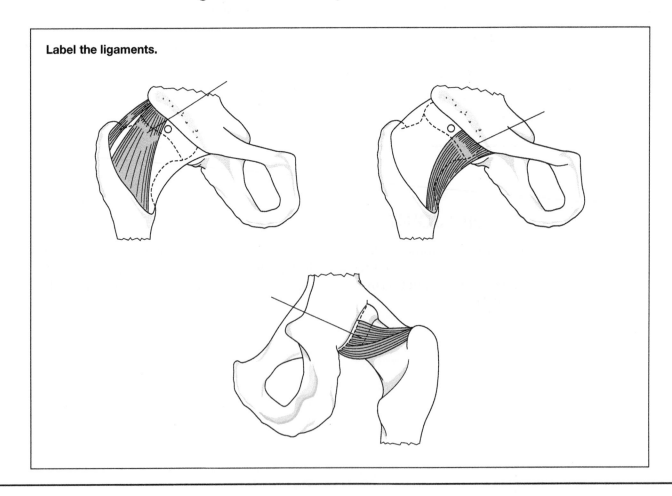

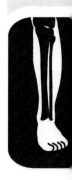

Professor says

On the above, label the following ligaments and add notes on their attachments below.

Iliofemoral ligament
(this is the strongest ligament in the body)
Attachments

Function

Pubofemoral ligament
Attachments

Function

Ischiofemoral ligament
Attachments

Function

Professor asks

What would happen if a ligament became:

1. Too lax?
2. Too tight? (contracted)
3. Snapped completely? (ruptured)
4. Became inflamed or torn?

Answer tips
1. Joint instability as is seen in degenerative joint diseases like osteoarthritis, for example, where joint space is diminished, resulting in the ligament effectively becoming too long to stabilise the joint.
2. Loss of joint mobility.
3. Major joint instability – oddly enough this is not always as painful as one might expect and may not be immediately diagnosed.
4. Torn ligaments cause pain on stressing of the ligament, local tenderness on palpation and may cause joint effusions (swelling confined to a joint cavity).

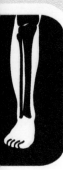

More on the hip joint

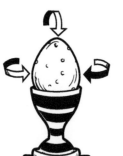

Shaped rather like an egg in an eggcup, the hip joint is a ball-and-socket joint; it allows an almost infinite combination of movements yet keeps its stability.

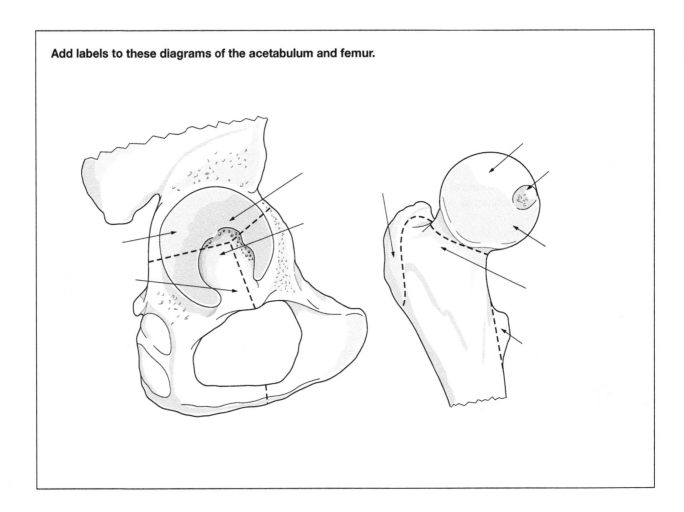

Add labels to these diagrams of the acetabulum and femur.

When you come to learn about the shoulder, the arrangement is a little similar but in the shoulder the egg cup does not make such a good job of containing the egg!

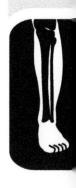

Professor says

Make your own notes on:

The Acetabulum

The Head of the Femur

The Acetabular Labrum

The Ligamentum Teres

The Articular Cartilages of the Femur and Acetabulum

The surface marking of the hip joint

How to locate the joint on a model. Find the mid-point of inguinal ligament, go 1.5 cm inferior, this corresponds to the surface marking of the anterior of the hip joint.

Have a go!

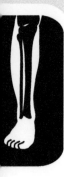

On these diagrams, draw the

acetabular labrum

inguinal ligament

obturator membrane

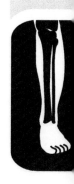

Movements at the hip

Table 2.1

Movement	Definition	Limiting factors to movement
Flexion		
Extension		
Abduction		
Adduction		
Internal (medial) rotation		
External (lateral) rotation		
Circumduction		

Note. Humans only have 10–15° of hip extension but loss of hip extension is bad news, it affects the push-off phase of gait and means that a person cannot stand with a normal erect posture. It does not really make as much of a functional impact if one loses a few degrees of hip flexion.

On your model and on the diagrams below locate the following:

Greater trochanter

Lesser trochanter (you cannot really palpate this on a model and it's probably best not to try, unless you want a slap!)

Adductor tubercle

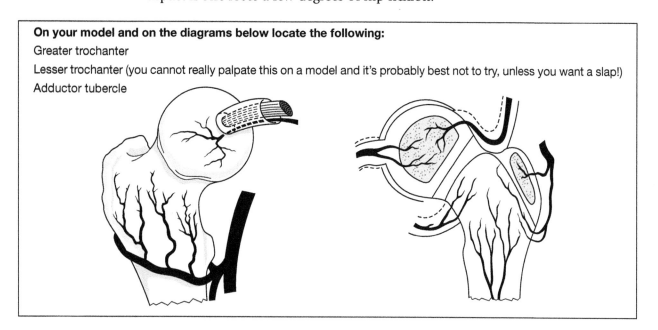

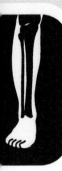

1. Where is the ligamentum teres and what does it do?
2. What deepens the socket of the hip joint?
3. Why does the femoral head sometimes die (avascular necrosis) following a badly displaced fracture or dislocation?
4. State two similarities and two differences between the hip and the shoulder joints.

Answers
1. The ligamentum teres is the internal ligament found within the hip joint. It might play a role in nutrition to the femoral head.
2. The labrum around the outer rim of the acetabulum.
3. The blood supply to the femoral head is complex, most blood supply is from the periarticular anastomosis – this may be disrupted following fracture of the neck of the femur. Hence the risk of avascular necrosis (death of the femoral head from lack of blood).
4. Two similarities – both possess a labrum, both are spheroidal.
5. Two differences – one has internal ligament, one has two necks (the humerus!).

THE PUBIC SYMPHYSIS

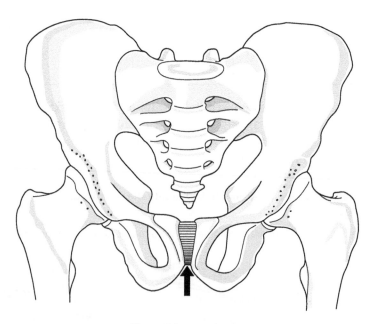

The pubic symphysis

The two pubic bones meet in the median plane at the pubic symphysis. It is a cartilaginous joint with a disc in between the bones.

☞ Suprapubic ligament
☞ Arcuate pubic ligament
☞ Movements (not much except during childbirth).

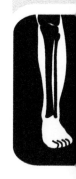

Give three factors that make the hip joint very stable:

1.

2.

3.

Clues: depth of acetabulum, shape of bones, ligaments, muscles.

Give three factors that make the hip joint very mobile:

1.

2.

3.

Clues: type of joint, lining of bones, shape of femoral neck.

Let's talk

It is important that you practise describing things verbally, this gets much easier with practice, it will help in your practical exams and when you treat patients. Get a watch with a second hand or a stopwatch. Ask a fellow student to time you for five minutes. Talk for the *whole* five minutes about the hip joint. Ask your friend to score you on:

☞ How interesting the talk was
☞ How accurate the talk was
☞ How much you hesitated
☞ How confident they would feel if they were your patient?

Do this twice. First of all, talk to your friend as though they were a patient who has asked you what a human hip joint is like. Remember, patients usually do not know any anatomy. Then repeat the talk as though you were talking to a lecturer who knows everything about the joint!
   Repeat this for

☞ the knee
☞ ankle joint
☞ the small joints of the foot

once you have learned about them.

THE THOMAS TEST

To test the right leg, perform passive hip and knee flexion on the opposite leg: a positive result occurs when the right hip flexes off the bed. Reason – at the extreme limit of hip flexion, the pelvis tilts posteriorly, i.e. the lumbar curve flattens.
   If there is sufficient extensibility in the anterior structures of the hip, the leg will remain on the bed; if not, it will rise off the bed.

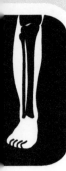

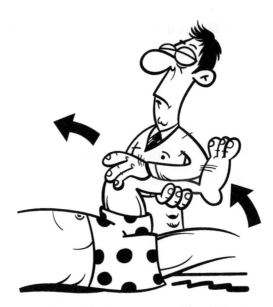

This is the Thomas test. The picture shows a positive result on the right leg. It is a test for a hip flexion deformity (contracture).

The other common test at the hip joint is the Trendelenburg test.

Do you know what this test demonstrates?

Answer
It is a test for weakness of the hip abductors – see 'gluteal gremlin' in the Muscles of the lower limb chapter.

Professor asks

Professor asks some typical anatomy questions

1. How does the structure of the hip joint relate to its function?
2. Give a detailed account of the muscles that abduct the hip and explain the signs and symptoms that result from weakness of these muscles.

Write a page on each of these.

What are the key words to underline?
What is the question asking?
What will the examiner be looking for?
What might be a common reason for some students to fail these type of questions?

THE KNEE JOINT

Get hold of a femur and a tibia and join them together as they would be in a living body (the most round part of the femoral condyles should be posterior, and the tibial tubercle should be anterior). Notice how they don't fit together as well as the femoral head did in the acetabulum at the hip joint. In fact if the knee only had bones to rely on for stability it would be very unstable! So what? Well, start thinking about what soft tissues might help the bones fit together a little better and give the knee joint some stability.

'Let's make a knee joint'

To help you understand some important concepts, we are going to make a knee joint. You will need two eggs, a saucer, doughnuts and some water.

1. Lay the saucer on a table – this represents the upper (superior) aspect of the tibia.

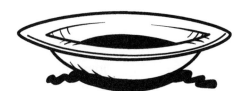

2. Put the eggs on top of the saucer – these represent the two femoral condyles at the lower end of the femur.

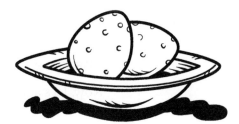

3. Notice how they roll around and end up lying on their side. This is because the radius of curvature of an egg is not uniform – now look at a real femoral condyle – the same applies, the posterior portion of the condyle is a smaller diameter sphere than the inferior part. This means that when the knee is in a flexed position, it is inherently unstable, but when extended, the flat part of the condyle is in contact with the tibia. This is more stable and close packed (we will come back to this term in a minute).

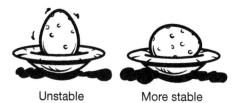

Unstable   More stable

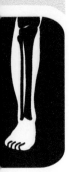

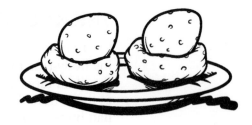

4. The problem is that the eggs still tend to roll around a little. So I now want you to put the two doughnuts on top of the saucer and rest an egg inside each. The doughnuts now represent the knee joint's menisci – they cradle the eggs, help them to become more stable and make the whole thing fit together better.

5. Now, if you wet the doughnuts to simulate synovial fluid and move the eggs around you will see that the doughnuts help more of the eggs' surface stay moist than the saucer alone could do. I know I'm rambling here but this is an important concept: articular cartilage relies on synovial fluid being swept over its surface to stay alive – this is called synovial sweep and it is another function of the menisci.

What does 'close packed' mean?

Joints have some positions in which they are more stable than others. The position of maximum stability is when there is maximum contact between the articular surfaces, and the surrounding ligaments are taut; this is close packed. Think of close packed as a pop bottle with the top screwed on tightly. So, for example, the knee is close packed when extended, and the ankle is close packed when dorsiflexed.

The bare bones

Now, let's add the collateral ligaments and the menisci.

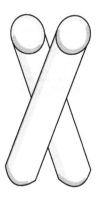

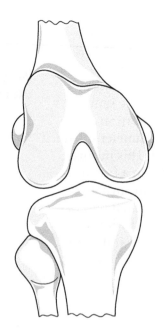

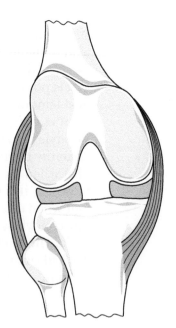

Now we add the cruciate ligaments.

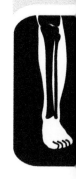

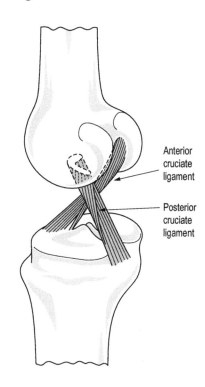

Location of anterior cruciate (ACL) and posterior cruciate ligaments (PCL).

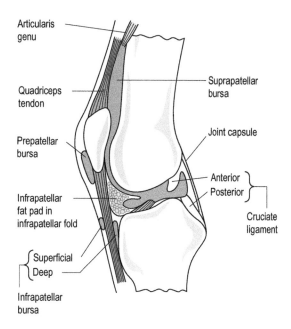

The patella. This is a sesamoid bone – a bone that is embedded within a tendon.

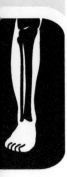

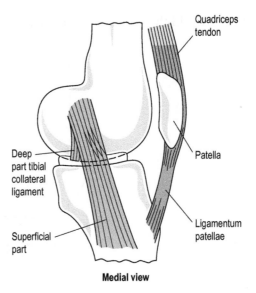

The medial tibial collateral ligament of the knee joint. Medial collateral ligament, a broad flat band, attached to medial meniscus so they may be injured together!

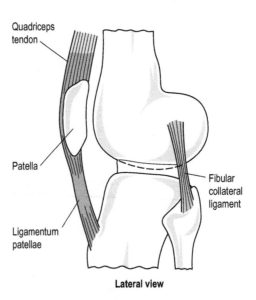

The lateral fibular collateral ligament of the knee joint.

Professor asks

Describe the medial and lateral collateral ligaments of the knee to a friend who knows nothing about anatomy, explain to your friend what their role is, how they differ and their similarities.

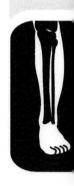

Table 2.2

Medial collateral ligament	Lateral collateral ligament
Attachments/Length	Attachments/Length
Shape	Shape
Function	Function
Relationship to medial meniscus	Relationship to lateral meniscus

Answer tips

Classical exam question here.

The lateral collateral ligament is cord-like and shorter than the medial collateral ligament and is not attached to the meniscus, unlike the medial collateral ligament.

Professor says

Complete Table 2.3.

Table 2.3

Medial meniscus	Lateral meniscus
Shape	Shape
Function	Function
Pathology	Pathology

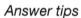

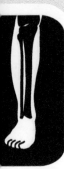

Answer tips

☞ Menisci are anchored to the tibia by coronary ligaments.

☞ Don't forget the menisci are not the same shape or size as each other.

☞ Medial is larger and semicircular.

☞ Lateral is smaller and more spherical.

☞ Functions = increase joint congruency.

☞ Assist in load bearing.

☞ Some shock absorption.

☞ Aid lubrication by facilitating synovial sweep.

☞ Assist in the locking mechanism of the knee.

☞ Menisci in cross-section.

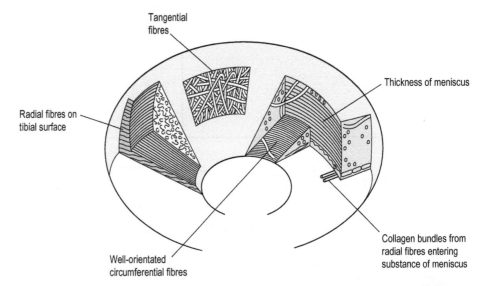

Diagram showing distribution of collagen fibres in the menisci of a knee.

Collagen is positioned in such a way as maximally to resist the forces brought to bear on the tissues. Most of the fibres are circumferentially arranged; a few are radially arranged, particularly on the tibial surface; these resist lateral spread of the meniscus. In the meniscus, tension is generated between the anterior and posterior attachments.

So what do the menisci do?

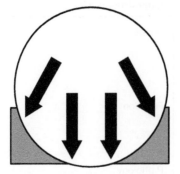

Menisci allow maximum contact between surfaces and spread of pressure

A

Menisci removed. Decreased congruency, decreased synovial sweep and loss of shock absorption

B

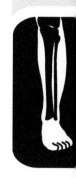

The menisci are shaped like two croissants, sat on the tibia, but one is more circular than the other. The croissants are bound onto the tibia by coronary ligaments (like a crown). The croissants help the femur to fit onto the tibia better, and they also help synovial fluid wash over the femoral condyles thus feeding them; this is synovial sweep.

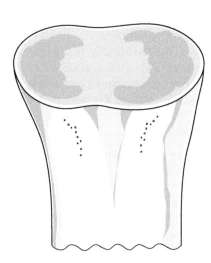

The croissant may tear along its length – longitudinal tear. If this happens, the loose flap lifts up like the handle on a bucket (bucket handle tear). It may also tear radially. Surgery to remove a meniscus is *menisectomy*. Peripheral tears of the meniscus may heal if sutured but sometimes it is just easier to remove the torn piece of croissant!

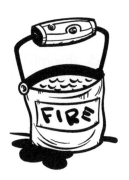

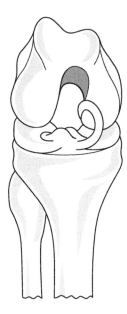

Professor says

Test yourself!

1. From what you have learned so far about the location, structure and function of the menisci, think of the symptoms that you might expect in a patient who has a torn meniscus.
2. Why do you think that the medial collateral ligament and medial meniscus are often injured simultaneously?
3. What is the relationship of the popliteus muscle to one of the menisci?
4. A patient who has sustained a ruptured anterior cruciate ligament runs a relatively high risk of sustaining a torn meniscus at a later stage – from what you have learned so far, hypothesise the reasons for this fact.

Answer tips

1. Torn meniscus 5 symptoms vary but possibly will complain of locking, giving way, recurrent effusions, loss of confidence, joint line tenderness, diffuse pain.
2. MCL and medial meniscus are connected therefore may be injured together.
3. Popliteus pulls the lateral meniscus out of the way during knee flexion; this might explain why it is injured less than its medial counterpart.
4. Ruptured ACL leads to abnormal knee biomechanics with increased shear forces on meniscus making it more liable to tear.

One of the functions of the menisci is to increase congruencey of the articular surfaces of the knee joint and to assist with synovial sweep (Aagaard and Verdonk 1999).

This sounds impressive, doesn't it, but what does it mean?

☞ Translate the statement into something which a patient with no anatomical knowledge could understand.
☞ Then repeat as if you were answering a written question or an anatomy viva.

The functions of the menisci are load transmission and shock absorption, based on their collagen architecture, biochemical fluid composition, and their proteoglycan-collagen framework.

Varus and valgus at the knee

Which is which? This often causes confusion – but not any more.

Just as there is air in between the varus knees, the word 'varus' has 'air' in the middle – sort of! Oh well, suit yourselves – I tried.

The term *genu* is sometimes used for the knee so you might come across the terms *genuvarus* and *genuvalgus*.

The anterior cruciate ligament

Attachments are from the posterior aspect of the medial surface of the lateral femoral condyle, to the fossa just anterior and lateral to the tibial spines. Recent work shows it to be made of three separate bundles, which are orientated to resist

Varus   Valgus

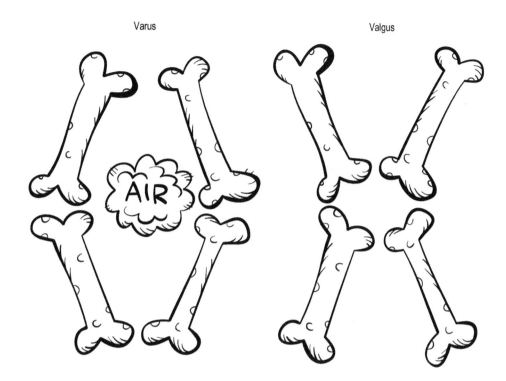

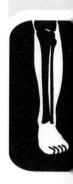

stresses from multiple directions. Its blood supply arises from the rich synovial fold which covers the ligament. One to 2% of the bulk of the ligament is neural tissue, containing Ruffini endings, Pacinian corpuscles, mechanoreceptors and free nerve endings. The proprioceptive role of the cruciates is vital.

Proprioception is the ability of the body to know its position in space.

Functions of the ACL

☞ It resists anterior tibial displacement on the femur.
☞ It prevents hyperextension of the knee.
☞ It controls and resists excessive rotation.
☞ It fine-tunes the locking mechanism.
☞ It acts as a secondary restraint against valgus and varus strain in all degrees of flexion.
☞ Major role in proprioception (Fischer-Rasmussen & Jensen 2000).

This is the PA draw test at the knee.

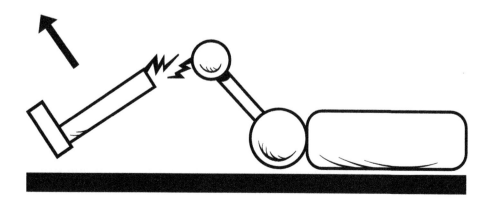

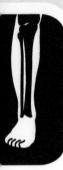

1. What does PA stand for?
2. What would you suspect if the tibia moved too much in the direction of the arrow?

Answers
1. Posterior anterior (pulling back to front).
2. Ruptured ACL.

The posterior cruciate ligament

Makris *et al.* (2000) discovered four functionally distinct groups of fibres within this ligament:

Anterior, Central, Posterior-longitudinal and Posterior-oblique.

The overall effect of the arrangement of these fibre bundles is that no matter what position your knee is put in, a portion of the ligament will always be under tension and therefore able to provide proprioceptive feedback and stability to the joint.

Attachments
From the depression in the intercondylar area of the tibia, it runs anteriorly, medially and proximally to the lateral surface of the medial femoral condyle.

Function (including) role in knee stability

Professor asks

What is proprioception?

Answer
Proprioception is the ability of your body to know where it is in space. For example, close your eyes and think about the position of your knee; you would be able to describe it very well without looking at it. Proprioception may be lost in some neurological or soft tissue conditions, causing tremendous problems.

The coronary ligaments

Location
These attach the menisci to the edge of the tibial condyles.

Function
They help to hold the menisci in place.

The transverse ligament

Function
Joins the anterior portion of the menisci together.

There are many other ligaments in the knee. And I will leave these up to you, But:

Make sure that you understand the functions and structure of the main four ligaments in the knee joint.

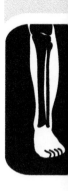

Prepare a summary of the tests that may be used to test the integrity of the ACL/PCL medial and lateral collateral ligaments.

Research the symptoms of patients who have ruptured (snapped) their anterior cruciate ligament – think about why they have each symptom. A pointer to get you started is that patients with a ruptured ACL lose proprioception in the affected knee joint (Fischer-Rasmussen & Jensen 2000).

Professor asks

What is a bursa?

Research three symptoms of bursitis (inflammation of a bursa).
Work out why each symptom occurs.
How would you describe a bursa to a patient?
What is housemaid's knee?

The patellar tap test
The knee has a large, expansive synovial membrane.

In injury or disease, one of the body's defence mechanisms is to produce more synovial fluid. If too much synovial fluid is produced it has nowhere to go except to float around inside the joint cavity. This is called an effusion. This is not the same as swelling which is not confined to a joint cavity.

If the effusion is large it can be seen (my knee swelled up like a football, Doctor!). If the effusion is less subtle, a test called the patellar tap test can tell you if there is a mild effusion.

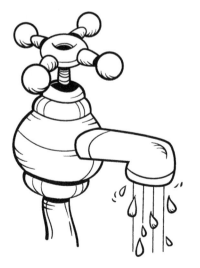
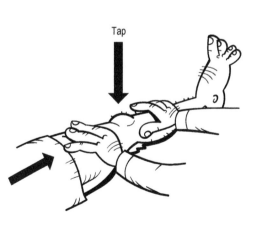

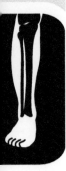

To perform the test, ask the patient to lie down, squeeze the fluid from the suprapatellar pouch (15 cm superior to the knee joint) by sliding your hand down towards the patella, and with your other hand bounce the patella on the femoral condyles. A tapping sensation or sound means there is an effusion.

Professor asks

1. What is oedema?
2. What is swelling?
3. What is effusion?

Answers
1. Oedema is an excess accumulation of tissue fluid in any part of the body, so it can be around the lungs for example – pulmonary oedema – or in the legs.
2. Swelling is a non-specific term that means something is bigger than it should be; this could include oedema, effusion, or things such as a tumour.
3. An effusion means that there has been a build-up of synovial fluid which remains contained within a joint capsule; for example after a sprained ankle.

Movements at the knee joint

The knee is not simply a hinge joint with flexion and extension, it also has rotation; students often forget this.

Sit in a chair with your feet on the ground and your knees at a right angle. Rotate your feet inwards and outwards – this is adjunct rotation at the knee – a

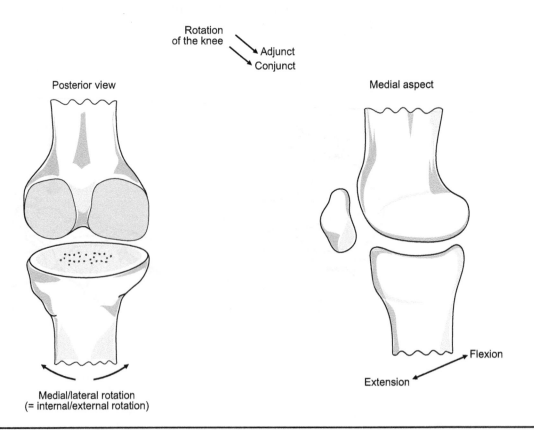

Rotation of the knee — Adjunct / Conjunct

Posterior view

Medial aspect

Medial/lateral rotation
(= internal/external rotation)

Flexion

Extension

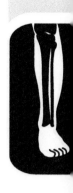

distinct movement that you do voluntarily. Don't forget that in anatomy you carry your syllabus around with you all the time if you need to check facts like this.

Now extend your knee joint until your leg is straight – believe it or not you have just performed conjunct rotation – straightening the knee is not a straightforward hinge movement. In the final 30° of knee extension, the tibia rotates laterally on the femur. This allows close packing or full congruency of the joint. This is an involuntary movement that occurs without your control. Because of the shape of the femoral condyles and the tension in surrounding ligaments this would also happen in a cadaver's leg. The other way of putting this is that the femur rotates medially on the leg if the foot is fixed on the ground. Because of this, you need a special muscle (popliteus) at the posterior of the knee to unlock it from full extension.

Remember *con*junct movement as your body is being *con*ned into rotating beyond its voluntary control.

Professor asks

Describe conjunct and adjunct rotation in the knee (as if you were doing a written exam, time yourself – 10 minutes).

Answer tips
Ten minutes is not long. Get the important concepts across with an example of each. The thrust of the answer should be that conjunct is an automatic, involuntary movement whereas adjunct is under voluntary control.

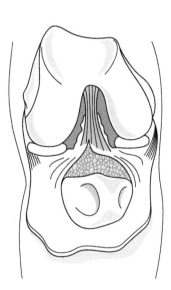

Inferior aspect of the femur, seen from below, and the posterior patellar surface

Occasionally, the patella does not track properly in the channel between the condyles of the femur; not surprisingly this is called a maltracking patella!

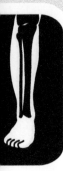

The knee – practical

Draw on your model:

☞ the medial and lateral femoral condyles (what is an epicondyle?)
☞ the medial collateral ligament
☞ the lateral collateral ligament
☞ the patella
☞ the patellar tendon (ligamentum patellae)
☞ the adductor tubercle
☞ the head of the fibula
☞ the tendon of biceps femoris
☞ there is a popliteal pulse behind the knee – it is not always easy to find, flex your model's knee to 45° and see if it is palpable.

Ligament tests in the knee joint

If your model has a known knee problem consult your lecturer before doing the tests below. There are many tests but these are the most important ones. You must be able to demonstrate the following tests:

☞ AP draw = PCL.
☞ PA draw = ACL.
☞ Varus stress test = LCL.
☞ Valgus stress test = MCL.

How would you …

a.   Test the integrity of your model's medial collateral ligament.

Your notes

_____

_____

b.   Test the integrity of your model's lateral collateral ligament.

Your notes

_____

_____

c.   Test the integrity of your model's anterior cruciate ligament.

Your notes

_____

_____

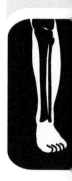

d. Test the integrity of your model's posterior cruciate ligament.

Your notes

_____

_____

e. What would be the significance of the following when these tests are carried out:
   1. Pain?
   2. Excessive movement?

Your notes

_____

_____

_____

_____

Answers
a. A valgus stress test.
b. A varus stress test.
c. A PA draw test (or also there is a Lachmans or pivot shift test).
d. An AP draw test.
e. 1. Pain means that some of the fibres of the ligament are torn
   2. Excessive movement means that there are many fibres torn or the ligament has snapped completely (ruptured).

☞ What four movements (in 2 planes) are possible at the knee joint?

Answer
1 Flexion, 2 extension, 3 medial lateral, 4 rotation.

Ask your model to perform them and carefully observe the muscles contracting.

☞ A fellow student is arguing with you; he says that the knee is a hinge joint. How do you convince him that he is wrong?
☞ What is conjunct rotation?
☞ What bony points can be palpated around the knee?

List them below.

_____

_____

_____

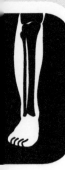

☞ Ask your model to lie down. Move your model's patella.

Questions about the patella:

1. In how many directions can it be moved?
2. Can the model do this voluntarily?
3. Why do we need a patella?
4. Can we live without a patella?

Answers:

1. It can be compressed, distracted, moved laterally, medially, superiorly and inferiorly.
2. No, the only movement that a person can do voluntarily is by flexing and extending the knee. Their patella will automatically track up and down, the other movements are what is known as accessory movements, i.e. they are important but you cannot do them on your own no matter how hard you try!
3. It makes the quadriceps work much more efficiently.
4. Yes.

Professor asks

What is the function of the menisci?

How many are there in each knee?

Draw the menisci below.
  from above
  in cross section

What are the differences between medial and lateral menisci?

Why do you need to know this?

Draw below two ways in which menisci might tear.

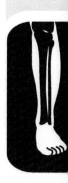

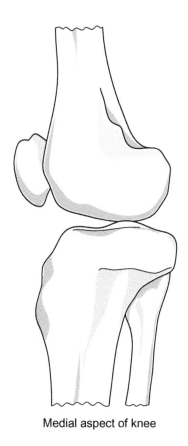

Medial aspect of knee

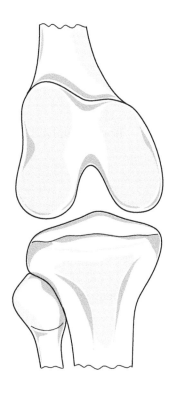

Anterior view of knee

To the above diagrams, add the:

cruciate ligaments × 2

collateral ligaments × 2

menisci × 2

Where would a fabella be?

Draw it on the diagram

What is a sesamoid bone?

Professor asks

1. Are the menisci palpable?
2. How are the menisci anchored to the tibia?
3. Why does the hip joint not require menisci?

Answers

1. The anterior margin may be palpated.
2. Coronary ligaments.
3. Bones themselves are congruent enough to make the joint stable, unlike the knee joint.

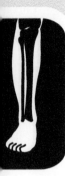

The menisci

The superior tibiofibular joint

Surface marking and joint line

Bones involved

Joint classification

Ligaments

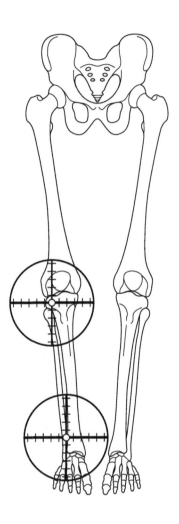

The inferior tibiofibular joint

Movements possible – some gapping occurs to permit final degrees of ankle dorsiflexion.

Professor says

Look at the problem at the top of the next page.

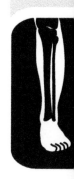

We make you study all this anatomy for a reason. Fred broke his ankle 6 months ago; the fracture was fixed surgically by placing a metal plate on the sides of his lower tibia and fibula (internal fixation). The fracture is now healed. The picture (right) shows you how the fracture has been fixed.

He comes to see you and is complaining that he cannot 'pull his foot up' (dorsiflex the ankle joint). (He has lost the final 5° of dorsiflexion when you measure his movements.)

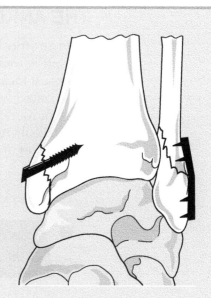

1. Using what you have learned about the tibiofibular joint so far, think of why this might be so.
2. Why has the medial malleolus been screwed back in place?
3. What would happen to the ankle joint if this had not been done?
4. What is an ORIF?

Answers

1. Final degrees of dorsiflexion are achieved by gapping of inferior tibiofibular joint.
2. Medial malleolus needs accurate reduction – reduction means aligning the bone ends after a fracture as it forms part of the ankle joint mortice.
3. Failure to fix this might result in an unstable ankle joint in the future and secondary osteoarthritis.
4. Open reduction internal fixation.

☞ How does the knee joint maintain its stability yet be able to move through a wide range of motion?
  Time yourself – 15 minutes to answer.
☞ How is the structure of the knee joint related to its function?
  Write a whole page of A4 on this.

Answer tips

If you are asked a question like this, do not just describe the structure and then describe the function – that is probably the commonest way to fail this type of question. Instead, link the two, e.g. the knee joint is a very mobile joint which is extended by the quadriceps muscle group – potentially at a mechanical disadvantage since it approaches the tibial tuberosity almost parallel to the femoral shaft. To minimise this, the knee joint has a patella to achieve a more efficient extension mechanism, changing the angle of approach of the quadriceps tendon.

Your turn!

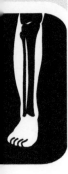

THE ANKLE JOINT

Hold an articulated (joined) foot in your hand. Look at the superior surface of the talus: it is wedge-shaped, fatter anteriorly, narrower posteriorly. This is relevant because it means that when the ankle is plantarflexed, the narrow part of the talus is in contact with the malleoli, allowing a large gap on either side and therefore more movement. When dorsiflexed, the wide part of the talus is locked between the malleoli, making it stable with almost no movement available; in fact the final few degrees of dorsiflexion are achieved by gapping apart of the tibia and fibula.

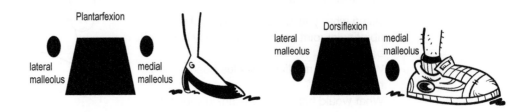

The collateral ligaments of the ankle joint

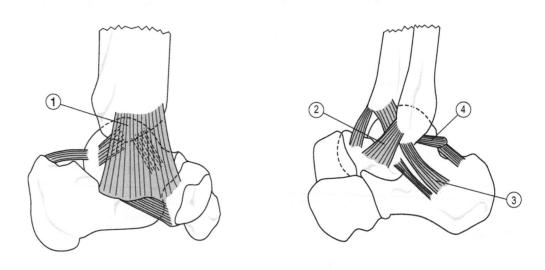

Therefore the closed packed position for the ankle is full dorsiflexion. The ankle is therefore less stable in plantarflexion and most injuries to the ligaments of the ankle occur when the foot is in some degree of plantarflexion (stiletto wearers beware!), e.g. when walking *down* stairs.

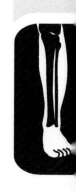

Summary – medial and lateral ligaments of the ankle joint:

Table 2.4

1 Deltoid	2 Anterior talofibular	3 Calcaneofibular	4 Posterior talofibular
Name	Name	Name	Name
Attachments	Attachments	Attachments	Attachments
Function	Function	Function	Function

Think about it, it makes perfect sense to put strong ligaments on either side of a hinge joint – if they were at the front and back they would interfere with movement and not resist lateral forces. Millions of years of evolution has done a pretty good job of preparing us for the stresses and strains which the body will have to endure.

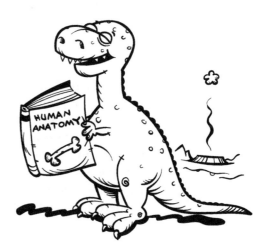

Remembering the lateral collateral ligaments at the ankle

Slide your hand down the outside of your leg, this more or less corresponds to the three lateral ligaments at the ankle joint.

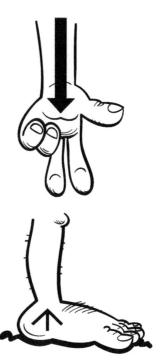

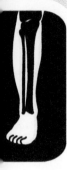

Professor asks

1. So, why does the hip joint not have two collateral ligaments?
2. You haven't done it yet, but if I told you that the elbow was a hinge joint, where would you put two ligaments?
3. What is an avulsion fracture?
4. Why are avulsion fractures common at the medial malleolus and not the lateral malleolus?
5. What does collateral mean?

Answers
1. Because it's not a hinge joint.
2. Either side of the joint.
3. Detachment of a piece of bone as a result of pull of associated ligament or tendon.
4. Deltoid ligament is very strong and so may pull off the tip of the medial malleolus, unlike the lateral ligament which will rupture first.
5. Either side.

This is where things get complicated (if they weren't already).

The ankle joint (talocrural joint) is between the tibia/fibula and the superior surface of the talus; it is a hinge joint allowing dorsi- and plantarflexion.

The talus sits on top of the calcaneus but not completely, so the calcaneus needs a scaffolding to *sustain* or hold the talus up. This is called the sustentaculum tali.

There is a joint on the underside of the talus between this and the superior surface of the calcaneus – the subtalar (talocalcanean) joint.

There are two points of contact here, anterior and posterior.

THE SUBTALAR JOINT

The joint has a concave posterior facet on inferior surface of talus and the convex posterior facet on the upper surface of the calcaneus.

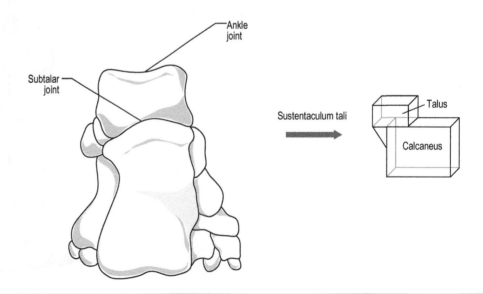

Movements at subtalar level (complicated)

Movement at the subtalar joint is often described as inversion and eversion. The triplanar motion of the talus occurs around a single axis, allowing components of pronation and supination to occur.

Think of the surfaces of the subtalar joint forming a cylinder whose long axis passes obliquely through the sinus tarsi.

Supination is calcaneal inversion + adduction + plantarflexion. **Pronation** is abduction + calcaneal eversion + dorsiflexion (remember prone to *bed* = *ab*duction *E*version *D*orsiflexion). Note that these movements all occur together and cannot be separated. Much gliding and rotation occurs at these two joints, by which the foot rotates underneath the talus. Inversion and eversion occur here. The axis for movement runs forwards, upwards and medially from the back of the calcaneus, through the sinus tarsi to emerge at the superomedial aspect of the neck of the talus.

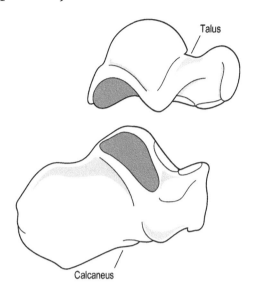
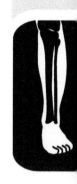

Talus

Calcaneus

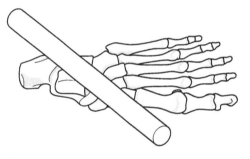

The axis of the subtalar joint

Describe the subtalar joint

☞ The bones involved.
☞ How they articulate.
☞ The ligaments involved
  – lateral talocalcanean
  – medial talocalcanean
  – interosseous talocalcanean
  – cervical
  – the axis of motion.

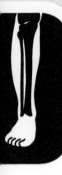

Draw on each other and on this diagram:

Greater trochanter

Head of fibula

Tendon of biceps femoris

Lateral collateral ligament of the knee

Tensor fasciae latae

Lateral malleolus

Peroneus longus

Peroneus brevis

Tubercle at base of 5th metatarsal

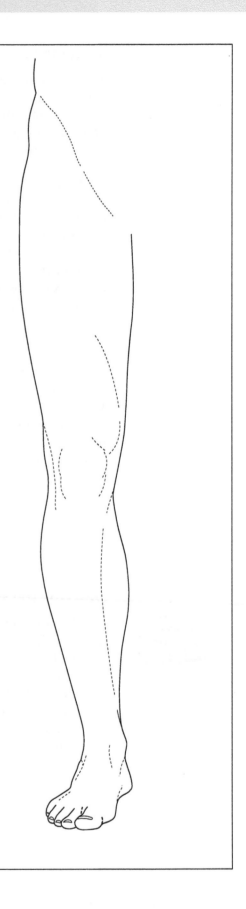

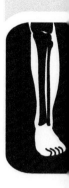

Draw the lateral ligaments of the ankle on this picture and on your model.

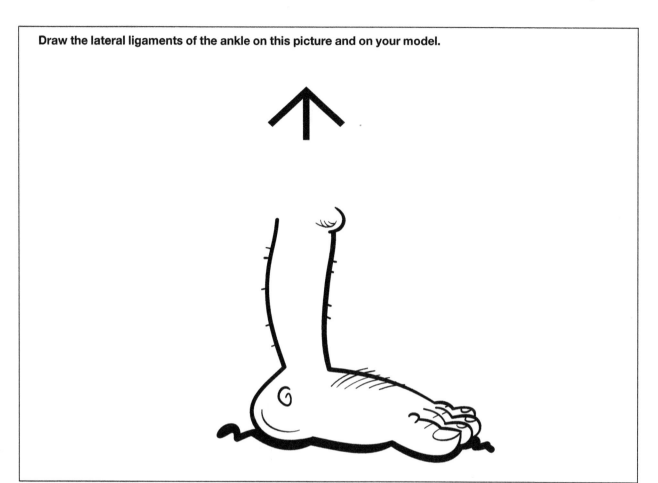

Draw the medial ligament (deltoid) of the ankle on this picture and on your model.

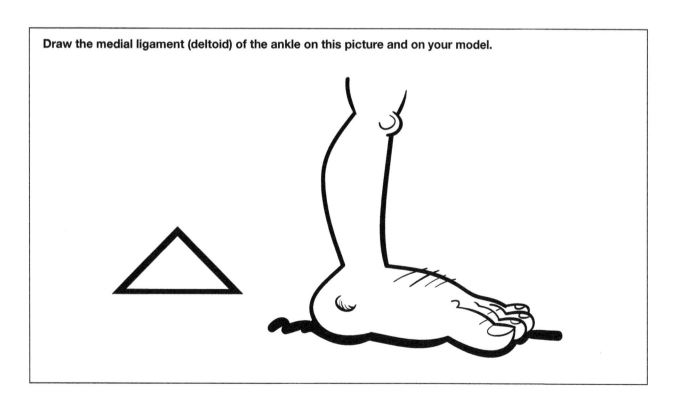

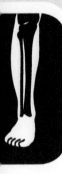

On this diagram and on your model, draw the:

medial and lateral heads of gastrocnemius

the musculotendinous junction

soleus

the Achilles tendon

tibialis anterior.

To this posterior view, add the bones which make up the ankle joint.

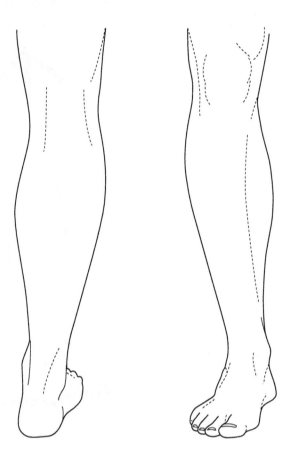

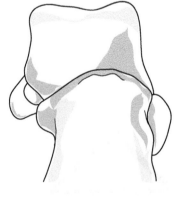

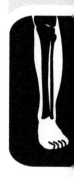

The ankle – practical

☞ On your model, draw the malleoli.
☞ Add the collateral ligaments.
☞ Dorsiflex your ankle and identify as many tendons as you can.
☞ Repeat and draw them on the leg of your model as they contract.
☞ Draw on your model the deltoid and lateral ligaments of the ankle.
☞ Draw on your model the retinaculae.
☞ What does retinaculum mean? What is their function?
☞ Draw on your model the plantar fascia – with care if they are ticklish.
☞ Draw the cuboid, tuberosity of navicular, neck of the talus, base of 5th metatarsal bone on your model.
☞ Draw the MTP joints, the IP joints and the head of the fibula on your model.
☞ Find the anterior tibial, dorsalis pedis and posterior tibial pulses on your model.

On your model, label the following:

☞ malleoli
☞ the tendons of extensor digitorum longus
☞ the tendons of extensor digitorum brevis
☞ extensor hallucis longus
☞ the retinaculae
☞ tendon of tibialis anterior.

If you are unsure about which tendon is which, ask your model to stand on one leg; their extensor tendons/dorsiflexors, etc., will work like crazy, especially if you make the model work by, for example, catching a ball.

On the diagrams and then on the leg of your model, draw the following:

The sustentaculum tali   Medial malleolus   Lateral malleolus   The three lateral collateral ligaments

Medial cuneiform   First metatarsal   The cuboid bone   Tuberosity at the base of the 5th

Deltoid ligament   Achilles tendon insertion   metatarsal

Medial view of ankle joint

Lateral view of ankle joint

MAKING IT REAL

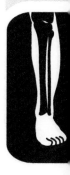

Anatomy should not be thought of as a textbook subject. It is probably the basis for the rest of your careers. I would like you to take a moment to think about why I ask you to learn anatomy in such great detail.

Look at these problems …

1. A patient comes to see you. He felt a 'twang' in the back of his leg yesterday when he was running to catch the bus. Passive SLR (straight leg raise) produces posterior thigh pain and so does resisted knee flexion; this is made worse by resisted lateral rotation of the knee.
   - Which muscle has he damaged?
   - How do you know?
   - What led you to your conclusion?
2. After a night clubbing you 'go over' on your ankle; you have forcibly inverted your ankle joint walking down some stairs:
   - Which ligaments have been stressed?
   - Which is the likeliest ligament to be damaged?
   - Why would this probably not have happened walking up stairs?
3. A friend stops you in the street. He has noticed a pain on the lateral side of his hip region following a long walk; he can feel a click when he swings his leg forwards and his leg aches around the greater trochanter area but he can move his hip fully with no pain. He is convinced that his hip is 'coming out of its socket'.

   From your knowledge of anatomy:
   - How can you be confident that this is unlikely?
   - What could be happening?
   - Is it relatively easy or hard to dislocate a hip joint? (not a hip replacement)

Answer 1
☞ Biceps femoris.
☞ Work it out – read Chapter 3.
☞ All resisted actions of the muscle are painful.

Answer 2
☞ Lateral ligament complex.
☞ Anterior talofibular ligament.
☞ Dorsiflexed ankle = close packed = more stable.

Answer 3
☞ It is very difficult to dislocate a healthy hip joint, it takes major trauma to do so, a car crash for example.
☞ What could be happening is iliotibial band syndrome, caused by overuse or inflammation of the iliotibial band.
☞ Very difficult – go and watch a hip replacement!

Talocalcaneonavicular joint (TCN)

This joint is between the ovoid head of the talus and concave posterior of the navicular, and the middle and anterior facets of the talus on the calcaneus. The spring

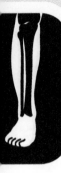

ligament (plantar calcaneonavicular) also contributes to this complex joint. Together with the calcaneocuboid joint these two joints form the junction between hindfoot and midfoot.

The calcaneocuboid joint

Your notes

_____

_____

_____

_____

_____

_____

The cuneonavicular joint

Your notes

_____

_____

_____

_____

_____

_____

The cuboidonavicular joint

Your notes

_____

_____

_____

_____

_____

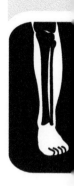

The tarsometatarsal joints

Your notes

_____

_____

_____

_____

_____

_____

_____

The intermetatarsal joints

Your notes

_____

_____

_____

_____

_____

_____

The metatarsophalangeal joints

Your notes

_____

_____

_____

_____

_____

_____

The interphalangeal joints

Your notes

_____

_____

_____

_____

Joints of the foot – a summary

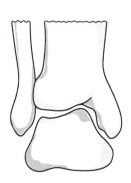

The ankle (talocrural) joint

= hinge joint

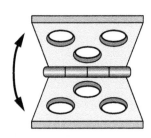

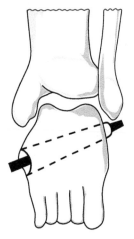

Subtalar (talocalcaneal) joint

complex, oblique axis

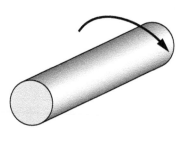

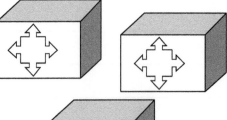

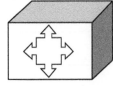

Intertarsal joints

plane joints, a small amount
of gliding occurs here

Label and classify the foot joints on this diagram.

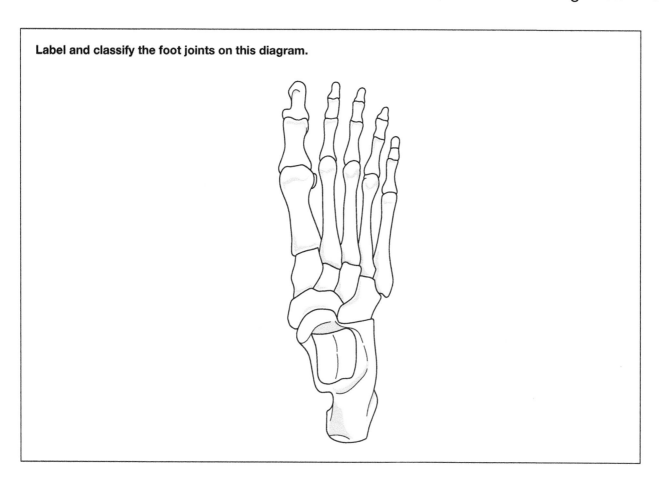

Here, I have separated the bones of the foot so that you can add your own notes on the joints if you wish.

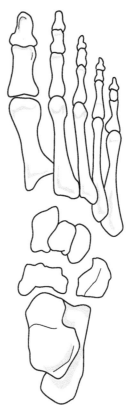

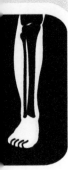

The plantar fascia:

Where is it?

What is its function?

What are its attachments?

The arches of the foot:

List them

Describe their structure

How are they maintained?

The retinaculae of the leg:

Where are they?

What is their function?

What are their attachments?

Long and short plantar ligaments:

Where are they?

What is their function?

What are their attachments?

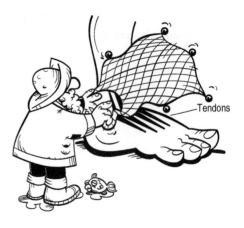

Tendons

LIMITING FACTORS

The soft tissue parts of a joint that may limit movement ligament, capsule, tendon, muscle, meniscus.

Bone to bone contact may limit movement – elbow extension, for example.

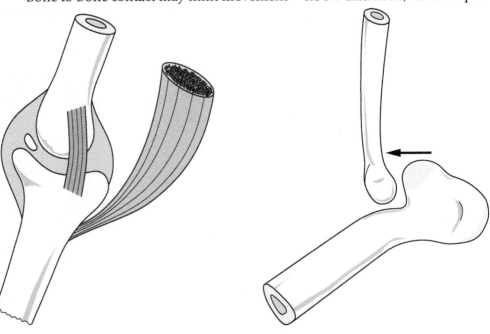

Unfortunately, sometimes our soft tissues get in the way, e.g. hip flexion.

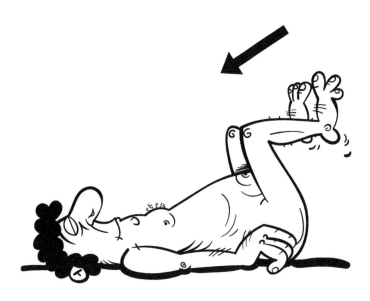

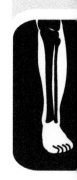

You need to know what *should* limit movement in a normal joint before you can tell what is abnormal.

Before your written and practical examinations, go through each of these points; can you write about each in detail and demonstrate it practically?

Table 2.5

Joint	Limiting factors in a normal joint
Hip	
Flexion	Soft tissue (abdomen!)
Extension	Iliofemoral ligament + hip flexors
Medial rotation	Lateral rotators, posterior capsule, ischiofemoral ligament
Lateral rotation	Lateral rotators, lateral band iliofemoral ligament
Abduction	Abduction medial band iliofemoral ligament
Adduction	Adductors, ligamentum teres, lateral band iliofemoral ligament
Knee	
Extension	Both collaterals, posterior capsule, skin, fascia, hamstrings, gastrocnemius, parts of both cruciates, anterior menisci (squeezed)
Flexion	Parts of both cruciates, posterior menisci (squeezed), quadriceps, anterior capsule soft tissue approximation
Ankle	
Dorsiflexion	Achilles tendon (if knee is extended)
	Posterior deltoid ligament
Plantarflexion	Calcaneofibular ligament
	By dorsiflexors
	Anterior deltoid ligament
	Anterior talofibular ligament

JOINTS

Hip

☞ Joint line.
☞ Movements.
☞ Limiting factors to movement.
☞ Bones involved.
☞ Classification.
☞ Three capsular ligaments/ligamentum teres.

Knee

☞ Joint line.
☞ Movements.
☞ Limiting factors to movement.
☞ Bones involved.
☞ Classification.
☞ Anterior and posterior cruciate ligaments.
☞ Medial and lateral collateral ligaments.
☞ Other ligaments less important, e.g. transverse, arcuate popliteal ligament, etc.

Patellofemoral joint and superior and inferior tibiofibular joints

☞ Palpate location.
☞ Joint line.
☞ Classification.
☞ Ligaments.

Ankle

☞ Joint line.
☞ Movements.
☞ Limiting factors to movement.
☞ Bones involved.
☞ Classification.
☞ Three lateral ligaments.
☞ Medial (deltoid) ligament.

Subtalar

☞ Movements.
☞ Limiting factors to movement.
☞ Bones involved.
☞ Classification.
☞ Ligaments.

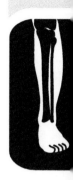

Intertarsal and tarsometatarsal joints

(Less detail needed)
☞ Bones involved.
☞ Classification.
☞ Movements possible.
☞ Main ligaments.

Metatarsophalangeal and interphalangeal joints

☞ Bones involved.
☞ Classification.
☞ Movements possible.
☞ Main ligaments.

Judgement time

It is now time for you to assess whether or not you have achieved the learning outcomes at the start of this chapter. You need to be able to tick each of these boxes. If you cannot, return to the relevant section of the chapter.

❑ Can you describe (for your written paper and orally for your exams) the structure of all joints of the lower limb including articular surfaces, movements possible, ligaments, capsule and other important features particular to that joint?

❑ Can you describe (for your written paper and orally for your exams) the function of all joints of the lower limb?

❑ Could you relate 1 (above) to 2 (above)?

❑ Do you have a working knowledge of limiting factors to movements of the joints of the lower limb?

❑ Can you demonstrate the surface marking of hip, knee, ankle, subtalar and midtarsal joints?

Muscles of the lower limb

Learning outcomes

After reading this chapter you should be able to describe the:

1. Origin.

2. Insertion.

3. Action.

4. Functional (applied) anatomy.

5. Nerve supplyof the muscles in this chapter.

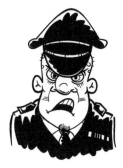

First of all, learn these important terms and don't argue!

☞ **Concentric:** muscle contraction which results in the muscle becoming shorter.
☞ **Eccentric:** when a muscle gradually controls movement by slowly lengthening – paying out length.
☞ **Isometric:** when there is no change in muscle length, e.g. a bodybuilder posing.
☞ **Reciprocal lengthening:** as a set of muscles work concentrically, the opposite muscles have to lengthen to allow movement otherwise we would never move anywhere!
☞ **Reciprocal shortening:** as a set of muscles work eccentrically, the opposite muscles have to 'gather up the slack' but the muscle is not actively contracting.

Concentric … eccentric … What's that all about then?

This is a tricky concept. Once you grasp it it's not that hard but until you do it will cause you some problems.

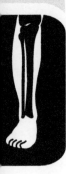

Here is my attempt to explain it.

Imagine a crane that has to lift a heavy weight. It does this by attaching a rope to it and winching up the rope. To lower the weight it still uses the same rope but the rope slowly pays out its length and gently lowers the weight to the floor.

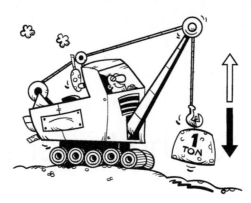

As the rope shortens the weight is pulled up = concentric contraction.

As the rope lengthens the weight is gently lowered = eccentric contraction.

MUSCLES AROUND THE HIP JOINT

Because the hip joint is a multi-axial joint (it can move in lots of directions), it needs many muscle groups to achieve and control movement. If it were a hinge joint it would only need flexors and extensors and your student life would be a lot simpler. In reality though, these are the groups of muscles that act at the hip joint:

☞ Flexors
☞ Extensors
☞ Abductors
☞ Adductors
☞ Lateral rotators
☞ Medial rotators.

All the above work in combination to produce circumduction – where the foot would trace out a cone.

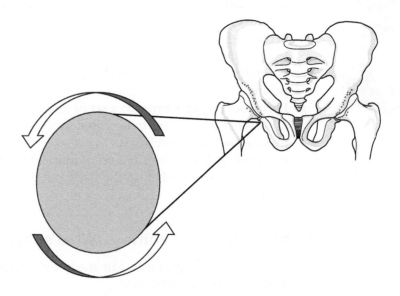

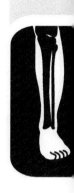

Table 3.1 Hip flexion

Muscle	Origin	Insertion	Nerve supply
Psoas major	transverse processes of L1–L5 vertebral bodies of T12–L4 and intervertebral discs	lesser trochanter	ventral rami, L1,2,3
Iliacus	inner surface of iliac fossa	insertion: lesser trochanter of the femur	femoral nerve, L3,4
Rectus femoris	straight head: anterior inferior iliac spine (AIIS) reflected head: ilium just above the acetabulum	tibial tuberosity	branches of femoral nerve, [L2],3,4
Sartorius	anterior superior iliac spine (ASIS)	upper medial surface of tibia	branches of femoral nerve, L2,3

Psoas and iliacus are too deep to palpate. Sartorius is the body's longest muscle and although not often injured it is used in many movements, especially when sitting cross-legged (the word 'sartorial' means to do with tailoring, this is how tailors used to sit). To demonstrate its action, imagine you had stepped on a drawing pin or something smelly in the street, and lift your foot up to look at the sole of your own foot – this is what sartorius does.

Professor says

Test yourself
On this picture, find the following muscles:

☞ Psoas major
☞ Iliacus.

Iliacus + psoas are sometimes called the iliopsoas.

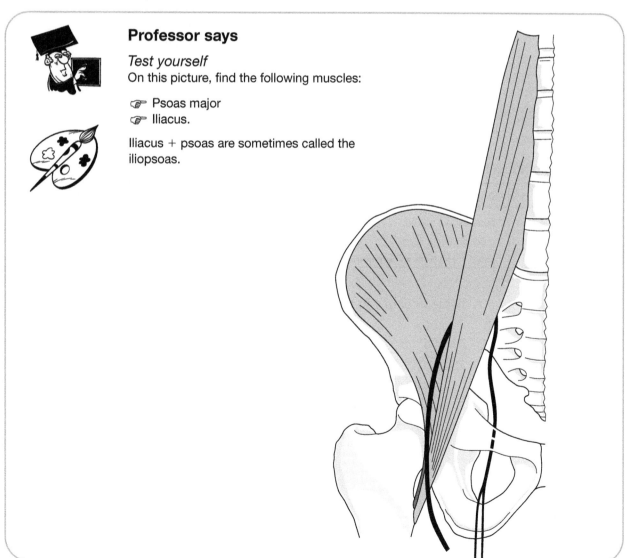

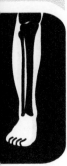

☞ Psoas major has the potential to stabilise the lumbar spine (Santaguida & McGill 1995).

☞ Muscle imbalance affecting the muscles of the hip joint is now thought to be one cause of low back pain (Nadler et al. 2001).

Table 3.2 Hip extension

Muscle	Origin	Insertion	Nerve supply
Gluteus maximus	outer rim of ilium, dorsal surface of sacrum and coccyx, sacrotuberous ligament	2 sites; 1. iliotibial band, 2. gluteal tuberosity on femur	inferior gluteal nerve, L5,S1,2
Biceps femoris	long head: ischial tuberosity short head: lateral lip of linea aspera	head of fibula	long head – tibial nerve, L5,S1,2 Short head – common peroneal nerve, L5,S1
Semitendinosus	ischial tuberosity	medial aspect of tibia contributes to the pes anserine	tibial nerve
Semimembranosus	ischial tuberosity	medial tibial condyle	tibial nerve

Gluteus maximus is the bulkiest muscle in the body.
It also helps to control knee stability – but how does it do this?
Clue: only some of its fibres attach to the femur.

Answer
Seventy-five percent of its fibres attach to the iliotibial band which crosses the knee joint and therefore can have a stabilising effect on it.

Table 3.3 Hip abduction (and medial rotation)

Muscle	Origin	Insertion	Nerve supply
Gluteus medius	outer aspect of ilium	greater trochanter	superior gluteal nerve
Gluteus minimus	outer aspect of ilium	greater trochanter	superior gluteal nerve
Tensor fasciae latae	anterior iliac crest anterior superior iliac spine	anterior aspect of IT band	superior gluteal nerve

A rhyme to help you to remember the hip abductors and medial rotators:

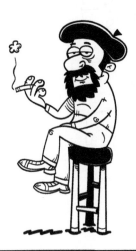

Tensor fasciae latae, gluteus med and min, all abduct the femur,
and rotate it in.

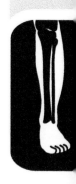

Table 3.4 Hip adduction

Muscle	Origin	Insertion	Nerve supply
Adductor longus	anterior surface of pubis	medial lip of linea aspera	obturator nerve, L2,3,4
Adductor brevis	body & inferior ramus of pubis	linea aspera	obturator nerve, L2,3
Adductor magnus	anterior fibres: inferior pubic ramus oblique fibres: ischial ramus posterior fibres: ischial tuberosity	proximal 1/3 of linea aspera adductor tubercle	anterior fibres: obturator nerve, L2,3,4 posterior fibres: tibial nerve of sciatic bundle, L4,5
Pectineus	pectineal line, superior pubic ramus	the pectineal line of the femur	femoral nerve, L3,4 OR obturator nerve, L2,3,4 OR femoral L3,4 and accessory obturator L3,4
Gracilis	pubic ramus	medial surface of proximal tibia contributes to the pes anserine	obturator nerve, L2,3,4

How to remember the hip adductors: 3 ducks peck at the grass
(hip adductors = 3 ad**duc**tors, **pec**tineus and **gra**cilis)

Table 3.5 Hip lateral rotation

Muscle	Origin	Insertion	Nerve supply
Quadratus femoris	lateral aspect of ischial tuberosity	quadrate line	nerve to quadratus femoris, L4,5,S1
Piriformis	pelvic surface of sacrum	medial surface of greater trochanter	nerve to piriformis, S1,2
Obturator internus	obturator foramen obturator membrane	medial aspect of greater trochanter	nerve to obturator internus, L5,S1,2
Obturator externus	obturator foramen obturator membrane	trochanteric fossa	obturator nerve, L2,3,4
Gemellus superior	ischial spine	medial aspect of greater trochanter	nerve to obturator internus, L5,S1,2
Gemellus inferior	ischial tuberosity	medial aspect of greater trochanter	nerve to quadratus femoris, L4,5,S1

These six muscles are all too deep to palpate. They are rarely injured so don't spend long hours worrying about them.

☞ Hip medial rotators.
☞ Gluteus minimus.

See the previous table on these muscles. The medial rotators also abduct the hip – saves you some revision at least!

Psoas and iliacus are stretched during lying prone.

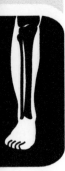

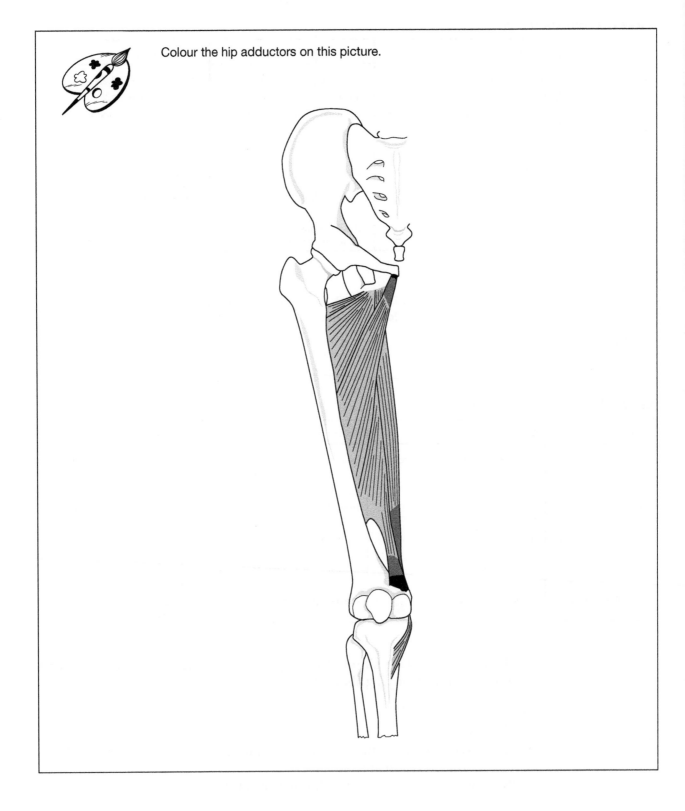

Colour the hip adductors on this picture.

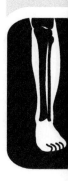

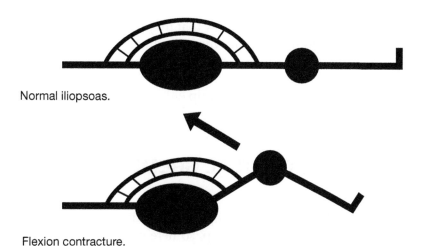

Normal iliopsoas.

Flexion contracture.

If there are soft tissue contractures in these muscles or the anterior of the hip capsule, lying or prone lying is painful or impossible – see Thomas test.

Most people with chronic back pain find lying flat uncomfortable because psoas also attaches to the lumbar spine and pulls on its spinal attachment in lying.

Gluteus maximus works hard when rising from a sitting position and extending the hip joint during push-off phase of walking.

If you have a patient on long-term bed rest, don't forget that these muscles atrophy (weaken) very quickly.

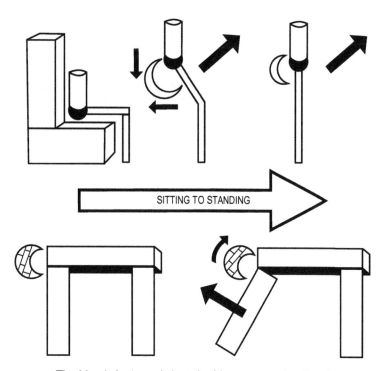

SITTING TO STANDING

The hip abductors abduct the hip – no surprise there!

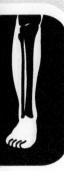

But – did you know that they also prevent adduction of the hip and prevent the pelvis from falling when standing on the same leg? If they are too weak to do this, the pelvis drops – see Trendelenburg sign.

You could think of the pelvis as a plank balanced on top of a golf ball (femoral head). The plank can tip either way, the hip abductors help control the plank!

THE GLUTEAL GREMLIN

The Trendelenburg sign is quite a difficult concept to grasp, so here goes with a really silly demonstration. I don't care that it is silly as long as it helps you to work it out. If it does not, please do not think any less of me, I'll be OK!

First of all imagine that the picture below represents the pelvis and hip joint.

As you can see, if you stood on your right leg, the left side of your pelvis can fall or rise pivoting upon the femoral head.

Now meet Gerald who will act out the role of gluteus medius and minimus for this demonstration.

See if this little guy helps you to understand the role of the hip abductors in maintaining a level pelvis.

Gerald is the Gluteal Gremlin. He has a rope in his hand and his bottom is glued to the greater trochanter. Because he is so strong, he pulls on the rope and keeps the weight level.

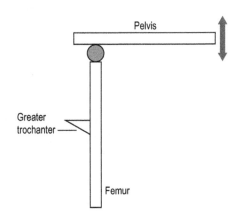

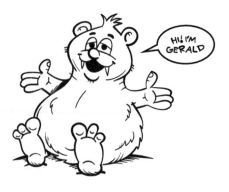

If someone suddenly cut the rope, the bar would dip to the opposite side – thus.

This is what happens when the hip abductor muscles are weak. They allow the opposite side of the pelvis to dip.

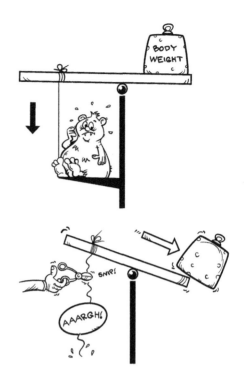

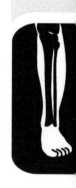

HUNG UP ON ACTIONS/ORIGINS AND INSERTIONS?

Do not forget that whilst a muscle has an action, e.g. flexion, it also resists the opposite movement. For example, biceps flexes the elbow but it can also prevent elbow extension, the hip abductors abduct the hip but they can also prevent adduction.

So what? Just because the anatomy books say that a muscle is an abductor, doesn't mean that all day long it abducts and does nothing else. How often do you actually abduct your hip during the course of a normal day? It is far more likely that you will use the abductors to prevent adduction as shown above. Never forget that functional anatomy is extremely important, i.e. how things actually work in a living body.

Imagine that you have been set the following exam question:

Give a detailed account of the muscles that abduct the hip joint and explain the signs and symptoms that would result from weakness of these muscles, and state how weakness of these muscles can be assessed clinically.

Answer on a page.

The other important test that you need to understand at the hip is the Thomas test. This is a test for a hip flexion deformity. Make notes below on:

How to perform the test.
What the test demonstrates.
What a positive result looks like.
You could be asked to demonstrate this in your practical exam.

Note that the Thomas test does not test for the strength of the hip flexors – it is a test of their length. Students often get this confused.

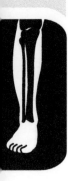
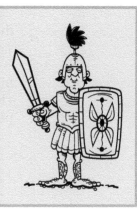

Gluteus maximus – practical

And no, gluteus maximus was not a Roman general or a gladiator!

Find the muscle on this picture, colour it in and then draw it on your partner.

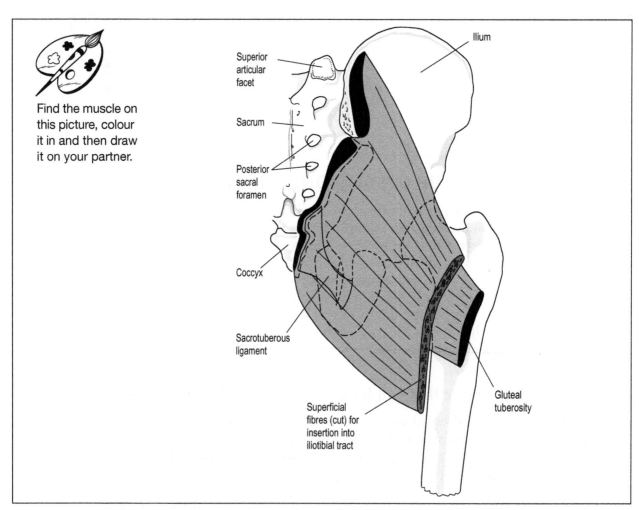

Questions
1. In which direction do its fibres run?
2. Demonstrate its functional activity.
3. Not all of its fibres attach to a bone; 75% of them in fact do not attach to bone, where do they attach?
4. Why do you need to know this?
5. Why do injections in this muscle have to be carefully placed?
Clue: what nerve passes deep to this muscle?

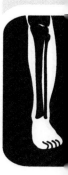

Answers
1. From superolateral to inferomedial.
2. Standing up from sitting down, or an activity involving hip extension.
3. 75% of its fibres attach to the iliotibial band.
4. Because I said so.
5. So you do not pierce the sciatic nerve.

Professor's tip

You would expect that a big sounding muscle would be supplied by a big sounding nerve, right? Well think again – gluteus *maximus* is supplied by the *inferior* gluteal nerve (remember a model thinking his or her *bottom* is *inferior*).

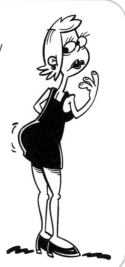

Hip abductors – practical

☞ How would a person walk if the hip abduction were weak?

☞ Demonstrate the gait to your partner.

☞ These two muscles insert onto the greater trochanter, so how can a forensic pathologist determine whether a skeleton belonged to a bodybuilder or a couch potato by looking at a greater trochanter and other bony lumps and bumps?

☞ Apart from hip abduction, what is the function of the hip abductors?
Answer: Medial rotation

☞ Is there a difference between medial and internal rotation?
Answer: No

☞ Is there a difference between external and lateral rotation?
Answer: No

☞ You are chatting to a patient who has had a total hip replacement. Their surgical incision goes through the gluteus medius and minimus – the patient is very concerned that when they walk, their operation leg tends to roll into external rotation and it is difficult for them to correct this. How do you explain this to your patient using your knowledge of anatomy?

Professor's tip

To palpate gluteus medius and minimus, stand with your legs slightly apart, place your hand above your greater trochanter but below your iliac crest, rock gently from side to side or stand on one leg – they contract strongly on the weight-bearing leg.

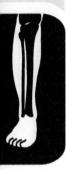

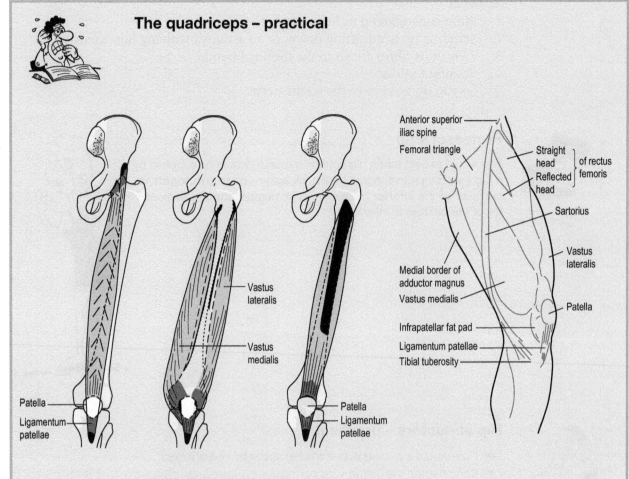

The quadriceps – practical

1. What does 'ceps' mean?
2. What does 'quad' mean?
3. List the component muscles of the quadriceps group below.
   (i)
   (ii)
   (iii)
   (iv)
4. Which is the odd one out and why?
5. Which one is too deep to palpate?
6. How does the patella ensure that the quadriceps can work effectively?

Answers
1. Head.
2. Four.
3. Vastus intermedius, lateralis, medialis rectus femoris.
4. Rectus femoris because it acts across the hip joint or v medialis because of its oblique pull or intermedius because of its depth or lateralis because it has a letter L!
5. Intermedius.
6. Changes the angle of approach of the patellar tendon.

THE Q ANGLE

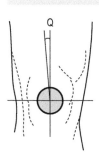

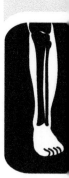

Exam tip – do not call them 'Quads' in exams and never use abbreviations unless you first define them.

On your model, draw a straight line across the middle of the patella. From the centre of this, draw a straight line going downwards through the centre of the tibial tuberosity, and another going upwards towards the ASIS.

This is known as the Q angle. It should be no more than 13° in males and no more than 18° in females – you will study this more in biomechanics.

Knowledge of this angle can assist with the diagnosis of patella maltracking.

The hamstrings – practical

Find the hamstrings on this diagram and colour them in.

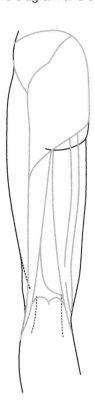

☞ How many hamstrings are there on each leg?
   Answer: 3
☞ On your model trace them from origin to insertion if possible. Why might this be difficult to do?
☞ Ask your model to lie prone and flex their knee to a right angle, then ask them to internally and externally rotate their leg.
☞ Which muscles are contracting during each part of the movement?
☞ Try this:
   – Sit with your knees extended (long sitting).
   – Try to touch your toes keeping your knees extended.

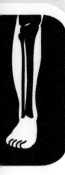

Now repeat this with your knees flexed.
– Why is it possible to go further if you flex your knees?
Answer: Muscles can stretch across one joint but not two simultaneously.

☞ What is the term for this phenomenon?
Answer: Passive insufficiency – the inability of a muscle to stretch maximally simultaneously across two joints.

☞ Why are hamstrings often injured?
Answer: They are two joint muscles.

☞ What is the action of the hamstrings at:
(i) The hip joint?
Answer: Extension (lies posterior to joint axis).
(ii) The knee joint?
Answer: Flexion (lies posterior to joint axis).
(iii) How do the hamstrings manage to perform rotation at the knee joint?
Answer: They attach on either side of the posterior aspect of the knee and thus have a rotary component.

Sartorius – practical

☞ What is the action of this long, strap-like muscle?
Answer: Hip flexion abduction lateral rotation

☞ How can you get your model to demonstrate sartorius at work?
Answer: Tell them they have just stepped on something smelly and wait until they look at the sole of their shoe!

☞ What does sartorial mean?
Answer: Connected with tailoring. Apparently tailors used to sit cross-legged

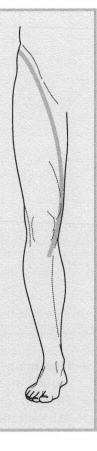

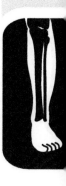

The hip adductors – practical

☞ On the inner (medial) thigh carefully find the tendon of adductor longus, the bellies of the adductors and the adductor tubercle.

☞ Ask your model to adduct against resistance and see which tendons can be palpated.

☞ Which of the hip adductors cross the knee joint?
Answer: Gracilis

☞ Why do you need to know this?
Answer: If it crosses the joint it might have an effect on its stability so don't forget it when you are treating knees!

How do I remember the names of the hip adductors?

Three ducks peck at the grass (please note that there is no grass though – they were really hungry!).

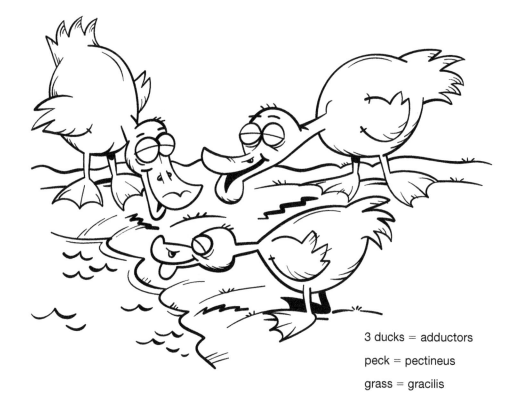

3 ducks = adductors

peck = pectineus

grass = gracilis

Two theories as to why I have drawn three ducks pecking at some grass:

1. I am working too hard and probably starting to lose it!
2. It is a good trick to help you to remember the names and numbers of the adductors of the hip joint.

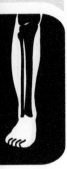

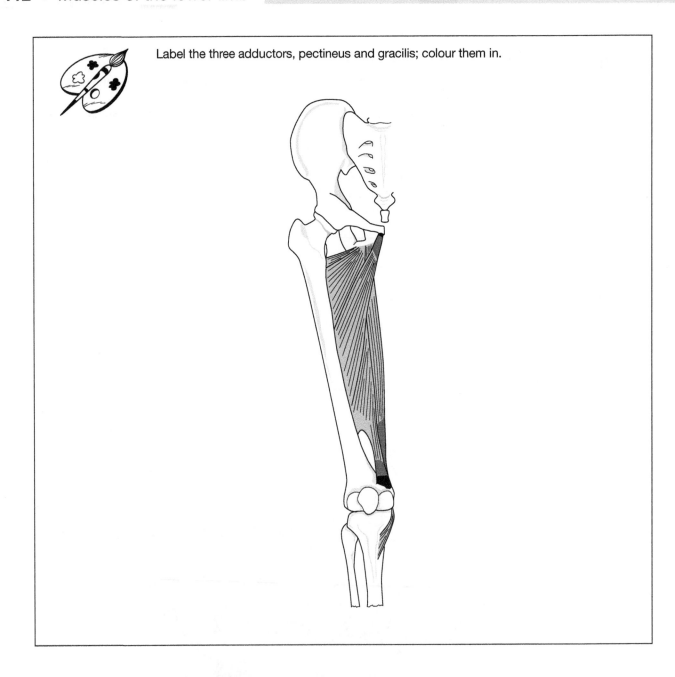

Label the three adductors, pectineus and gracilis; colour them in.

MUSCLES AROUND THE KNEE JOINT

These are:

☞ Flexors
☞ Extensors
☞ Lateral rotators
☞ Medial rotators.

There are others which cross the knee joint (therefore helping to stabilise it).

Table 3.6 Knee flexion

Muscle	Origin	Insertion	Nerve supply
Biceps femoris	long head: ischial tuberosity short head: lateral lip of linea aspera lateral tibial condyle	head of fibula	long head – tibial nerve, L5,S1,2 short head – common peroneal nerve, L5,S1
Semitendinosus	ischial tuberosity	medial aspect of tibia contributes to the pes anserine	tibial nerve
Semimembranosus	ischial tuberosity	medial tibial condyle	tibial nerve
Popliteus*	lateral femoral condyle arcuate popliteal ligament lateral meniscus knee joint capsule	posterior tibial surface	tibial nerve, L5,S1
Plantaris	above the lateral head of gastrocnemius on femur	medial to calcaneal tendon	tibial nerve, S1,2
Gastrocnemius	medial head: above medial condyle of femur lateral head: above lateral condyle of femur	calcaneus	tibial nerve, S1,2

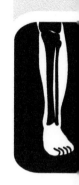

*Popliteus – the coolest muscle in the world! It is small but it does some great things:

1. It unlocks the knee from full extension (remember we said that the knee was not a hinge joint – popliteus proves that. Without a popliteus you could not unlock your knees – imagine that!
2. It pulls the lateral meniscus out of the way during knee flexion to protect it – bless it.
3. Its origin is inside the knee joint, so if you ever get a chance to go and see an arthroscopy you may get to meet one in the flesh! (Incidentally my second choice for world's coolest muscle would be articularis genus – look it up in this book.)

The muscles that flex the knee joint

How can I remember the muscles that flex the knee?
(Thanks to Marc Hudson, 1st year Physiotherapy student (class of 99).)

The muscles that flex the knee joint:

☞ Hamstrings*
☞ Gastrocnemius*
☞ Gracilis
☞ Sartorius
☞ Popliteus*

*main role

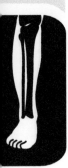

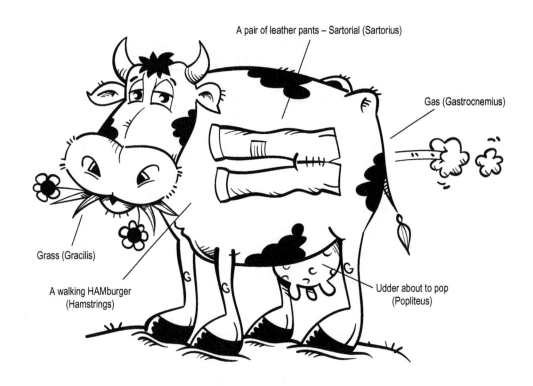

A pair of leather pants – Sartorial (Sartorius)

Gas (Gastrocnemius)

Grass (Gracilis)

A walking HAMburger (Hamstrings)

Udder about to pop (Popliteus)

Table 3.7 Knee extension

Muscle	Origin	Insertion	Nerve supply
Rectus femoris	straight head: anterior inferior iliac spine (AIIS) reflected head: ilium just above the acetabulum	tibial tuberosity via patellar ligament	Nerve: branches of femoral nerve, [L2],3,4
Vastus intermedius	anterior lateral aspect of the femoral shaft	tibial tuberosity via patellar ligament	branches of femoral nerve, [L2],3,4
Vastus lateralis	greater trochanter, linea aspera	tibial tuberosity via patellar ligament	branches of femoral nerve, [L2],3,4
Vastus medialis	intertrochanteric line of femur, medial aspect of linea aspera	tibial tuberosity via patellar ligament	femoral nerve, [L2],3,4
Articularis genus	distal portion of anterior femoral surface	synovial membrane of the knee joint	branches of femoral nerve, L3,4

useless fact number

3,567

There is a cute little muscle called articularis genus, which has been shown to perform a very important function. 'It elevates the capsule and the synovial membrane of the knee joint and prevents them from being pinched during extension of the leg' (Ahmad 1975).

So what?

So in theory, teaching a person with an immobilised knee joint (such as in a plaster cast) to do isometric quadriceps contractions will maintain the mobility of the synovium of the knee – it might be worth throwing that in to a practical exam or clinical placement sometime! Not a lot of people know that – now you do.

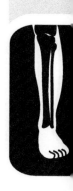

Pull the other one

Athletes often damage rectus femoris by extending the hip while simultaneously flexing the knee, e.g. kicking. Two joint muscles are frequently injured. Look at how vastus medialis pulls at a much more oblique angle than the other three 'quads' in an attempt to prevent the patella being pulled too laterally (see maltracking patella/chondromalacia/recurrent dislocation of patella).

Question

There is another clever mechanism, which exists to prevent this tendency of the patella to be pulled laterally, what is it?

Answer

The lateral femoral condyle has a bony ridge to keep the patella in check, sometimes this is underdeveloped, leading to problems such as recurrent dislocations of the patella.

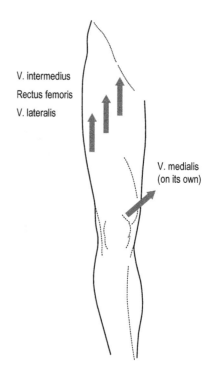

V. intermedius
Rectus femoris
V. lateralis

V. medialis (on its own)

Right knee – anterior view

How to remember some important sites of muscle insertions

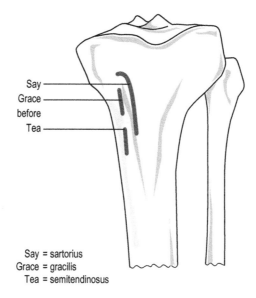

Say
Grace
before
Tea

Say = sartorius
Grace = gracilis
Tea = semitendinosus

This rhyme may help you to remember the insertions of these three muscles. This region is sometimes called the pes anserinus, and the associated bursa the pes anserinus bursa.

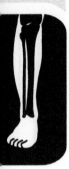

Injury to the hamstrings

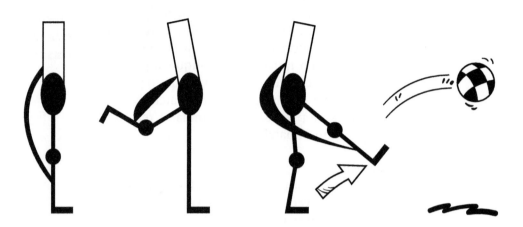

The hamstrings are posterior to the hip and knee joints so they flex the knee and extend the hip. If they are fully stretched over both hip and knee at the same time as in, for example, hurdling, or striking a football, they may tear. The inability to stretch across both joints at once is known as passive insufficiency.

MUSCLES AROUND THE ANKLE JOINT

These are

☞ Dorsiflexors
☞ Plantarflexors
☞ Invertors
☞ Evertors.

(*Note*: extrinsic muscles have origins in the leg but insertions in the foot.)

Table 3.8 Ankle dorsiflexion

Muscle	Origin	Insertion	Nerve supply
Tibialis anterior	lateral tibial condyle, proximal 2/3 of anterolateral surface of tibia	base of 1st metatarsal, medial cuneiform	deep peroneal nerve, L4,5,S1
Extensor hallucis longus	medial aspect of the fibula interosseous membrane	proximal and distal phalanx of hallux	deep peroneal nerve, L4,5,S1
Extensor digitorum longus	lateral condyle of the tibia upper anterior surface of fibula	dorsal surface of the bases of the middle & distal phalanxes of the 2nd–5th rays	deep peroneal nerve, L4,5,S1
Peroneus tertius (not everybody has one of these – don't worry, you'll live without one!)	distal 1/3 of anterior fibula	base of 5th metatarsal	deep peroneal nerve, L4,5,S1

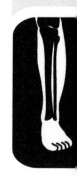

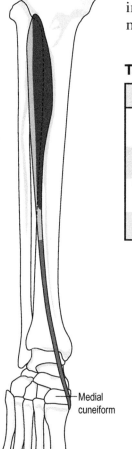

Medial cuneiform

Tibialis anterior acts as a brake to decelerate the foot following heel strike in walking. If tibialis anterior is not working (e.g. after injury to the common peroneal nerve), a foot drop occurs, this may be heard as the foot slaps on the ground.

Table 3.9 Ankle plantarflexion

Muscle	Origin	Insertion	Nerve supply
Gastrocnemius	two heads from above medial and lateral femoral condyles	calcaneus	
Soleus	upper fibula soleal line on tibia	calcaneus	tibial nerve, S1,2
Tibialis posterior	posterior tibia and interosseous membrane	navicular, all 3 cuneiforms, bases of 2–4 metatarsals	tibial nerve
Plantaris	above lateral head of gastrocnemius	medial to Achilles tendon or blended with it	tibial nerve

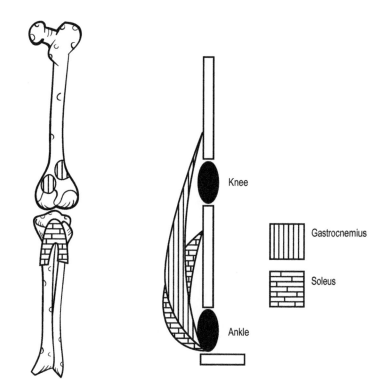

Knee

Gastrocnemius

Soleus

Ankle

Gastrocnemius is mainly fast twitch, soleus is mainly slow twitch. What does this statement mean? Make sure you understand the differences between type I and type II muscle fibres.

☞ What does gastrocnemius do that soleus does not?
  Answer: Flexes the knee
☞ Where does the Achilles tendon insert?
  Answer: Look it up, don't get lazy on me
☞ What is the triceps surae?
  Answer: Old term for gastrocnemius and soleus combined – 'sural' refers to the leg

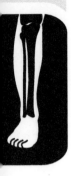

☞ What is a fabella?

Answer: A small sesamoid bone embedded in one of the heads of gastrocnemius; not everyone has one and it can appear like a loose body on a lateral knee X-ray.

☞ How can one diagnose a ruptured Achilles tendon?

Answer: Squeeze test/Thompson test. Lie the patient prone with their foot over the edge of the bed and squeeze their calf: no movement – ruptured tendon; slight plantarflexion – intact Achilles tendon. Once you know how – try the test on your model.

☞ What do you understand by the term musculotendinous (MT) junction?

☞ Draw the MT junctions of gastrocnemius on your model.

☞ On your model, draw the Achilles tendon.

More on gastrocnemius and soleus

On this diagram, label and colour the following:

Plantaris

Soleus

The Achilles tendon

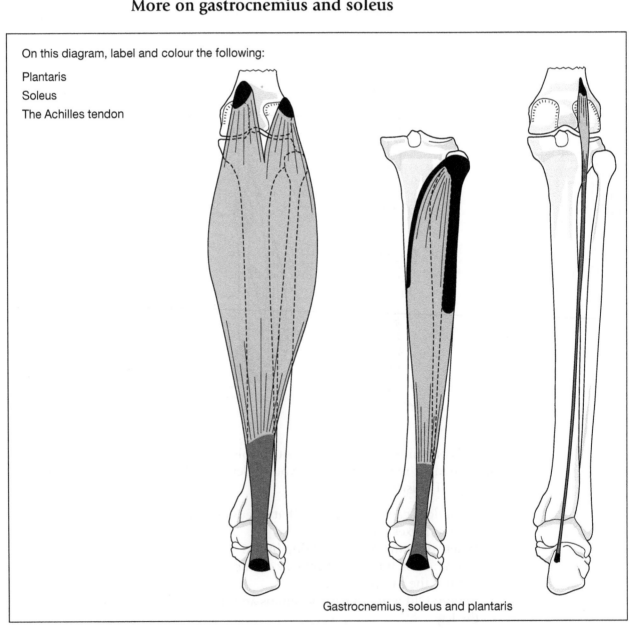

Gastrocnemius, soleus and plantaris

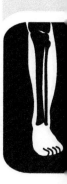

☞ On your model, demonstrate a functional activity of gastrocnemius and soleus.

☞ Find peroneus longus and brevis.

☞ Find the Achilles tendon.

Table 3.10 Inversion

Muscle	Origin	Insertion	Nerve supply
Tibialis anterior	lateral tibial condyle, proximal 2/3 of anterolateral surface of tibia	base of 1st metatarsal, medial cuneiform	deep peroneal nerve, L4,5,S1
Tibialis posterior	posterior, proximal tibia interosseous membrane medial surface of fibula	navicular tuberosity, all 3 cuneiforms, bases of 2nd–4th metatarsals, cuboid, sustentaculum tali	tibial nerve, L5,S1

Table 3.11 Eversion

Muscle	Origin	Insertion	Nerve supply
Peroneus longus	head of the fibula proximal 2/3 of lateral fibula	base of 1st metatarsal medial cuneiform	superficial peroneal nerve, L4,5,S1
Peroneus brevis	distal 2/3 of lateral fibula	base of 5th metatarsal	superficial peroneal nerve, L4,5,S1

The peronei

These muscles often cause confusion amongst students. They are evertors of the foot and plantarflexors of the ankle.

Professor asks

Q. Why do they evert the ankle?

A. Because they are on the lateral aspect of the leg.

Q. Why do they assist plantar flexion?

A. Because they pass behind the lateral malleolus and therefore are posterior to the ankle joint.

How do I remember the peronei?

Imagine a pair of knee-high boots. Sounds like per-o-ne-i. The zip on the outside of the boot corresponds to the location of the peronei.

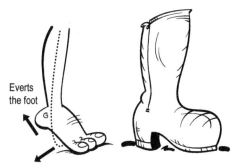

Everts the foot

Plantarflexes weakly

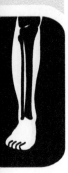

Professor's tip

Students very often get mixed up between the muscles supplied by the deep and superficial peroneal nerves. Here are two alternative methods that will help, one for the boys, one for the girls!

GIRLS. You get back from the shops after having purchased your designer 'peroknee' high boots (above) and your flat-mate accuses you of being very superficial (thus you remember that the *peronei* are supplied by the *superficial* peroneal nerve).

BOYS. Your bank manager refuses you a loan so you stand face on to him and kick him in the *shins* causing a *deep* bruise (not that I advocate violence). Thus you remember that the *anterior* tibials are supplied by the *deep* peroneal nerve.

Biomechanical research by Hunt *et al.* (2001) suggests that peroneus longus has an important role to play in causing eversion after heel contact in the gait cycle. It acts to stabilise the forefoot after heel rise, whereas peroneus brevis seems to have a role in preventing lateral rotation of the leg over the foot later on in the stance phase of gait.

What do the retinaculae do?

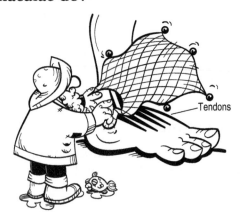

Table 3.12 Toe extensors and flexors

Muscle	Origin	Insertion	Nerve supply
Extensor hallucis longus	medial aspect of the fibula interosseous membrane	proximal and distal phalanx of hallux	deep peroneal nerve, L4,5,S1
Extensor digitorum longus	lateral condyle of the tibia upper anterior surface of fibula	dorsal surface of the bases of the middle and distal phalanxes of the 2nd–5th rays	deep peroneal nerve, L4,5,S1
Flexor hallucis longus	posterior, inferior 2/3 of fibula	distal phalanx of hallux	tibial nerve, L5,S1
Flexor digitorum longus	posterior surface of tibia	plantar surface of bases of the 2nd–5th distal phalanges	tibial nerve, L5,S1

Intrinsic muscles of the foot (the four layers)

(Intrinsic muscles, i.e. they have origin and insertion within the foot.)

Muscle

Superficial layer

Abductor hallucis

Flexor digitorum brevis

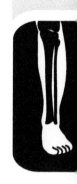

Abductor
digiti
minimi
Middle layer
Tendon of flexor hallucis longus (fhl)
Tendon of flexor digitorum longus (fdl)
Flexor digitorum accessorius
Lumbricals
Deep layer
Flexor hallucis
brevis
Adductor hallucis
brevis
Interosseous layer
Plantar interossei
Dorsal interossei

Revision layer aids: remember the words DAB and PAD. Dorsal Abduct DAB Plantar Adduct PAD (note – same applies in the hand).

Revision poetry

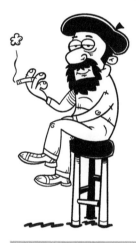

Medial plantar nerve supplies, Abductor Hall 'neath which it lies,
Flexors brevis, dig and Hall and the first lumbrical.

Judgement time

Let's assess whether or not you have achieved the learning outcomes at the start of this chapter.

You need to be able to tick each of these boxes. If you cannot, return to the relevant section of the chapter.

Can you now describe in writing and verbally the:

❑ Origin

❑ Insertion

❑ Action

❑ Functional (applied) anatomy

❑ Nerve supply

of the muscles in this chapter?

4

Nerves of the lower limb

Learning outcomes

After reading this chapter you should be able to describe

1. Root level.

2. Relations.

3. Major branches.

4. Innervations.

5. Signs and symptoms resulting from lesions of the nerves listed below:

   - Sacral and lumbar plexuses
   - Sciatic nerve
   - Common peroneal nerve
   - Superficial peroneal nerve
   - Deep peroneal nerve
   - Tibial nerve.

6. Obturator and femoral nerves – gross structure and location only.

7. The dermatomes of the lower and upper limbs.

THE SACRAL PLEXUS

The term 'plexus' refers to a network of nerves or blood vessels. The nervous system features a number of these networks, where autonomic and voluntary nerve fibres join together. These networks include the brachial plexus (shoulder), the cervical plexus (neck), the coccygeal plexus (coccyx) and sacral or lumbosacral plexus (lower back).

THE SCIATIC NERVE

The sciatic nerve (largest in the body) branches off the spinal cord between the fourth lumbar and third sacral vertebrae (L4, 5, S1, 2, 3). It extends down

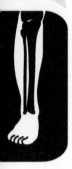

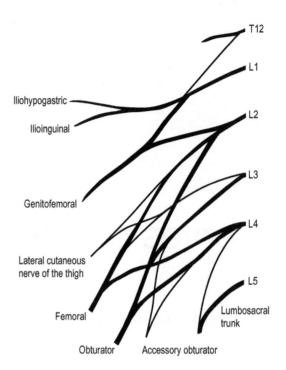

The lumbar plexus

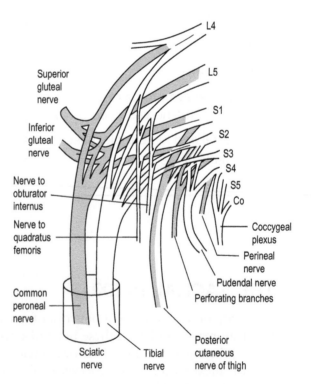

The sacral plexus

the centre of the posterior of the thigh. It appears as one single nerve until it reaches the apex of the popliteal fossa when it splits into two, the common peroneal and tibial nerves (remember though that strictly speaking it has always been two distinct nerves from the gluteal region). It innervates the hamstrings. Inflammation of the sciatic nerve, a condition known as sciatica, is a common

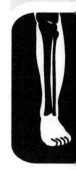

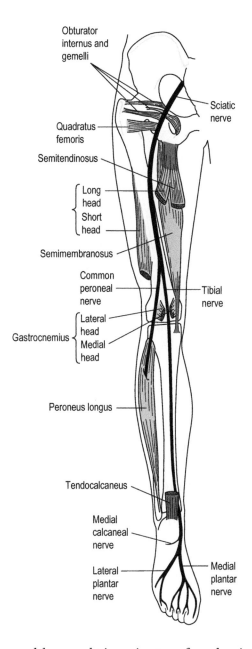

Obturator internus and gemelli

Sciatic nerve

Quadratus femoris

Semitendinosus

{ Long head
Short head }

Semimembranosus

Common peroneal nerve

Tibial nerve

Gastrocnemius { Lateral head
Medial head }

Peroneus longus

Tendocalcaneus

Medial calcaneal nerve

Lateral plantar nerve

Medial plantar nerve

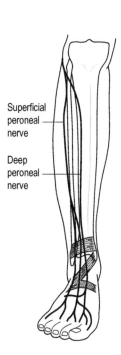

Superficial peroneal nerve

Deep peroneal nerve

problem and gives rise to referred pain (pain felt in a place other than where the actual problem is).

The tibial nerve branches off the sciatic nerve and, distally, divides into anterior and posterior branches. These branches innervate the muscles of the lower leg, ankle and foot.

The peroneal nerves include the common, superficial and deep peroneal nerves. Originating in the sciatic nerves, which branch off the spinal cord between the fourth lumbar and third sacral vertebrae, these nerves extend to the calf muscles, the skin of the top of the foot, and the toes.

The common peroneal nerve can often be palpated as it winds around the neck of the fibula; it may be compressed by a plaster cast which is too tight, and this may cause a foot drop – why?

Also, it is at exactly the same height as the bumper on a car – so it is quite vulnerable to being damaged.

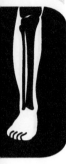

THE FEMORAL NERVE

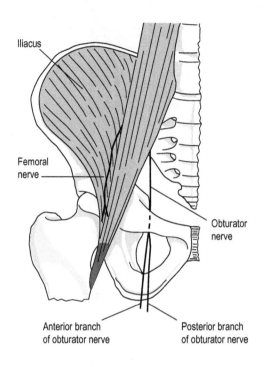

The femoral nerve branches off the spinal cord between the second and fourth lumbar vertebrae (L2, 3, 4). It extends down the anterior of the thigh to supply the muscles and skin of the leg, including the thigh, knee, part of the calf, the ankle and the foot.

DERMATOMES

A dermatome is the area of skin supplied by a particular nerve root level. Note that there are differences from one textbook to the next, and from one human to the next.

So what? Well, it is possible for two people to have damage to the same nerve root level, but to have different symptoms. Dermatomes are important as they can act as strong clues when you are attempting to make a diagnosis. Speaking from personal experience, I hurt my back several years ago and it resulted in sciatic pain, and pins and needles (paraesthesia) down the inside of my shin, including my big toe. I am confident that my problem occurred at L4 level. You also need to know the myotomes of the body (the same as above but this term relates to muscles supplied by a particular nerve root level). For example the quadriceps is supplied by L2, 3, 4 and 'C3, 4 and 5 keep the diaphragm alive'.

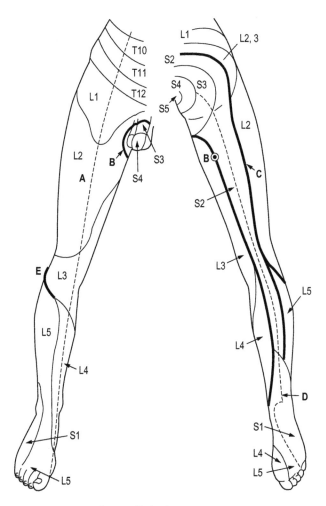

Lower limb dermatomes

Make sure that you understand the following:

1. Structure of a mixed spinal nerve
2. Function of a mixed spinal nerve
3. Dermatomes
4. Myotomes.

Complete a summary of the:

1. Functional
2. Motor
3. Sensory loss.

That would occur in the following scenarios:

1. A patient has their common peroneal nerve severed by a traffic accident at the level of the neck of the fibula.
2. A patient is stabbed in the popliteal fossa, completely severing the tibial nerve.

On these legs, draw the:

☞ sciatic
☞ obturator
☞ femoral nerves.

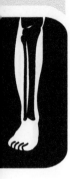

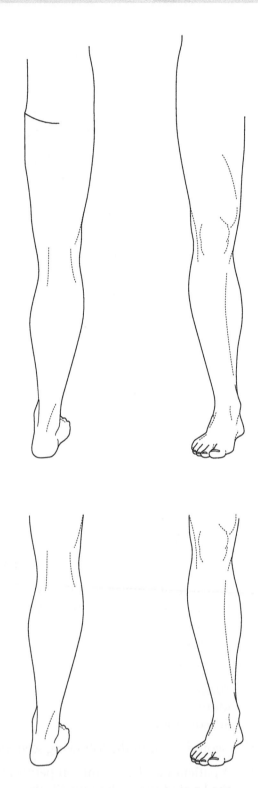

Now, draw the dermatomes of the lower limb on these legs.

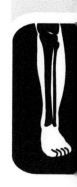

Judgement time

Check that you can describe

- ❑ Root level
- ❑ Relations
- ❑ Major branches
- ❑ Innervations
- ❑ Signs and symptoms resulting from lesions of these nerves
- ❑ Sacral and lumbar plexuses
- ❑ Sciatic nerve
- ❑ Common peroneal nerve
- ❑ Superficial peroneal nerve
- ❑ Deep peroneal nerve
- ❑ Tibial nerve
- ❑ Medial/Lateral plantar nerves

❑ Do you know the gross structure, root level and location of the obturator and femoral nerves?

❑ Do you know the dermatomes of the lower limb?

PART

2

Bones of the upper limb

Learning outcomes

After reading this chapter you should be able to:

1. Describe in detail the structure and function of all of the bones of the upper limb.

2. Be able to palpate these bony points (on two models of different gender).

   - Spine of scapula
   - Inferior angle of scapula
   - Acromion process
   - Acromioclavicular joint
   - Sternoclavicular joint
   - Coracoid process
   - Clavicle
   - Greater tuberosity of humerus

   - Medial and lateral epicondyles of humerus
   - Olecranon
   - Radial head
   - Ulnar styloid
   - Radial styloid
   - Pisiform
   - Hook of hamate
   - Metacarpals 1,2,3,4,5
   - Phalanges,1,2,3,4,5

3. Be able to identify the bony attachments of the muscles and ligaments listed in other chapters of this book

THE BARE BONES

The scapula

The scapula (shoulder blade) is more or less triangular in shape; with the clavicle or collar bone it forms the pectoral or shoulder girdle. The scapula has two thick borders, but if you hold one up to a bright light, the centre is so thin that it is translucent (allows light through).

Professor asks

Why is the central portion of the scapula so thin?

Answer
The central part does not need to be very thick, so it isn't! The medial and lateral borders have powerful muscle attachments, however, so the bone needs to be thicker here to withstand their daily pull.

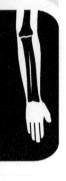

The humerus articulates with the scapula to form the shoulder or glenohumeral joint. This articulation takes place at the glenoid cavity, located at the upper, lateral angle of the scapula. The articular surface of the glenoid is about one-third the size of the articular surface of the humeral head. This is important to know because it means that from the bone point of view the shoulder joint is very unstable. We will need to add soft tissues later to make the shoulder more stable.

The posterior of the scapula features a laterally running line, which separates the surface into two unequally sized parts. This spine continues laterally and projects into the coracoid and the acromion (the acromion articulates with the lateral end of the clavicle). Both of these projections serve as anchors for muscle and connective tissue attachments; the spine and the acromion house the powerful trapezius and deltoid muscles. The shoulder joint and girdle are very mobile, but at the expense of some stability (it is much easier to dislocate a shoulder than a hip).

The shoulder joint may be considered as a mobile joint on a mobile platform, whereas the hip joint is basically a mobile joint on a fixed platform (the pelvis).

Add labels to these diagrams:

supraspinous fossa
infraspinous fossa
acromion

suprascapular notch
inferior angle
medial border

lateral border
coracoid process
glenoid fossa.

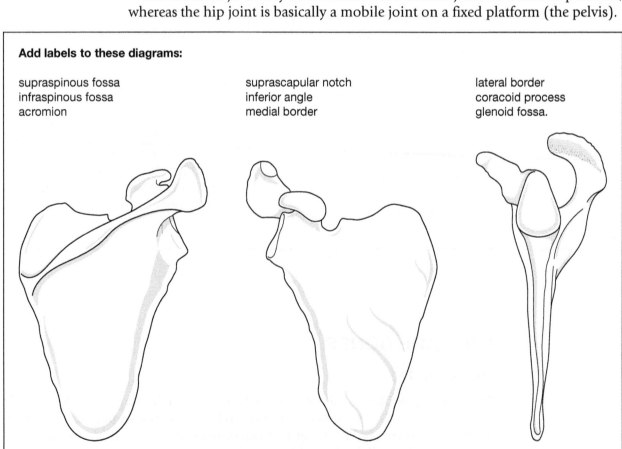

Many conditions and pathologies affect the shoulder: fractures, tendon and muscle problems, bursitis, etc. You need to fully understand the anatomy, function and biomechanics of the shoulder well in order to effectively diagnose and treat patients. Off we go (again!).

Label the following

coracoid process
acromion
infraglenoid tubercle
supraglenoid tubercle

lateral border
inferior angle
glenoid fossa.

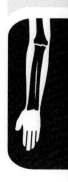

Professor asks

1. Which bones have an articulation with the scapula?
2. How is the stability of the scapula maintained?
3. What does supraspinous mean?
4. What does infraglenoid mean?

Answers

1. The clavicle and the humerus.
2. By soft tissues – muscles in particular.
3. Above the spine.
4. Below the glenoid.

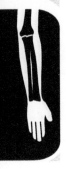

BONY POINTS AROUND THE SHOULDER

☞ Hold a scapula – describe it to your partner (partner – time how long it is before they run out of words).

☞ Hold a humerus – describe it to your partner (partner – time how long it is before they run out of words).

☞ Find and draw on your model:
- spine of scapula
- acromion
- coracoid
- greater tuberosity
- humerus
- sternum
- xiphoid
- medial border of scapula
- inferior angle of scapula
- medial and lateral humeral epicondyles.

THE CLAVICLE

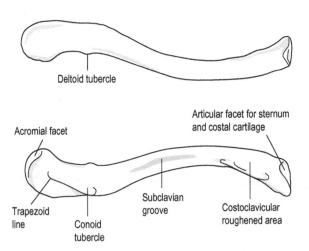

The clavicle or collar bone is a long, slightly curving bone which forms the anterior part of each shoulder girdle. Located above the first rib on each side, each clavicle attaches to the sternum medially and laterally. The clavicle joins with the acromion process to form the acromioclavicular joint (ACJ). The clavicle acts to brace the scapula and gives the shoulder girdle mobility and stability. It houses some important ligaments and is important in controlling the way in which the shoulder girdle moves (scapulohumeral rhythm).

THE HUMERUS

The humerus is the long bone of the upper arm. Its head is articulated with the scapula at the shoulder joint and its distal end articulates with the radius and ulna, forming the elbow joint.

Add labels

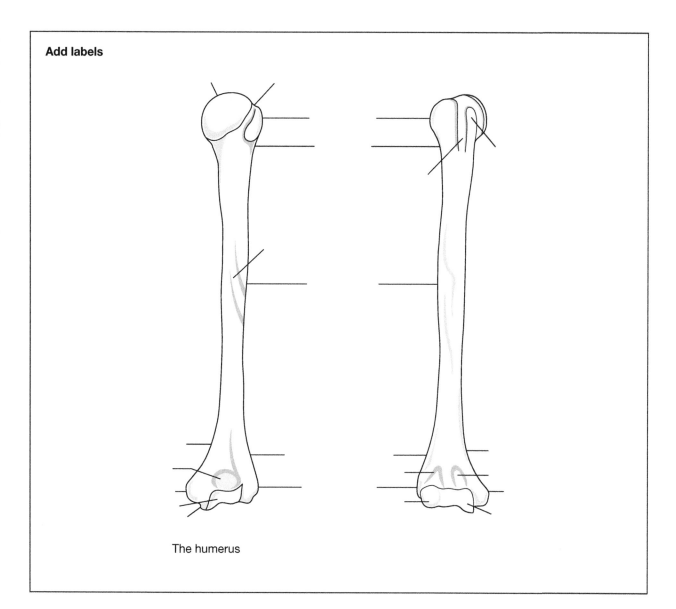

The humerus

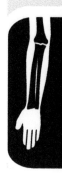

Professor asks

Which joint is at the proximal end of the humerus?
Which joints are at the distal end of the humerus?
In what ways are the humerus and the femur alike?
In what ways are the humerus and the femur different?

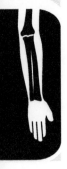

THE RADIUS

The radius is one of the two long arm bones (the other is the ulna) that form the forearm. The radius articulates at each end with the ends of the ulna, with the humerus at the elbow, and some of the carpal bones at the wrist. When the hand is turned with the palm facing up (supination) the radius is on the lateral side. When the hand is placed with the palm down (pronated) the radius crosses over the ulna in mid forearm.

THE ULNA

The ulna articulates at each end with the radius and with the humerus at the elbow. The ulna is always on the medial (little finger) side of the forearm.

ULNA
Olecranon
Trochlear notch
RADIUS
Head
Neck
Supinator crest
Radial tuberosity
Neck
Ulnar styloid process
Dorsal tubercle
Radial styloid process

HUMERUS

ULNA: fat at the top, thin at the bottom

RADIUS: thin at the top, fat at the bottom

DISC

Carpal bones x 8

How do I remember which bone articulates with which part of the humerus? The radius is so *radiant* that the humerus just **capitulates** and gives in (**radius = capitulum**).
The ulna is **un**believably stubborn and **tri**vial (**ulna = tro**chlea).

THE HAND

Each hand is made up of 27 bones. Eight of these bones form the compact arrangement known as the carpus. These carpal bones include two rows of four bones. The distal row articulates with the five metacarpals and the proximal bones articulate with the wrist joint. The long metacarpals form the broad structure of the hand and they in turn articulate with the phalanges.

The bones of the fingers are called phalanges (singular = phalanx) – the same as in the foot. Each finger has three phalanges, with the exception of the thumb, which has two. The end of each phalanx is bulbous at the site of articulation with other bones.

How do I remember the eight bones of the carpus?

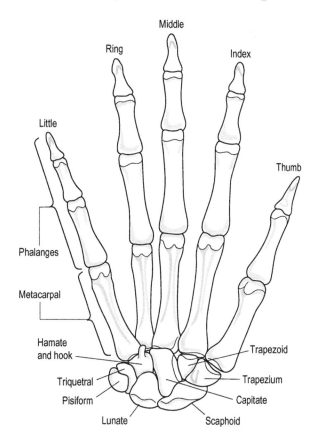
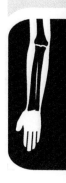

SIMPLY (scaphoid)	LEARN (lunate)	THE (triquetral)	PARTS (pisiform)
THAT (trapezium)	THE (trapezoid)	CARPUS (capitate)	HAS (hamate)

Another rhyme to remember the carpal bones!

Some	Lovers	Try	Positions
That	They	Can't	Handle

Your notes on the carpal bones

Scaphoid _____

Lunate _____

Triquetral _____

Pisiform _____

Trapezium _____

Trapezoid _____

Capitate _____

Hamate _____

The metacarpals

Draw them

Make notes on each

Classify the bones

The proximal phalanges

Draw them

Make notes on each

Classify the bones

Identify their palpable landmarks on a model

The intermediate phalanges

Draw them

Make notes on each

Classify the bones

The distal phalanges

Draw them

Make notes on each

Classify the bones

Look up the sesamoid bones in the hand

Judgement time

Theory
You need to be able to describe and identify all the features of bones included in this chapter.

Practical – bony points and landmarks

You must be able to find on a model the following:

- Clavicle (whole length)
- Acromion
- Coracoid process
- Head of humerus
- Radial styloid
- Ulnar styloid
- Posterior border of ulna
- Sternal notch
- Spine of scapula
- Inferior angle scapula
- Greater tuberosity humerus
- Medial epicondyle humerus
- Lateral epicondyle humerus
- Radial head
- Olecranon
- Head of ulna
- Metacarpals 1–5
- All proximal phalanges
- All terminal phalanges
- Pisiform
- Scaphoid
- Hook of hamate

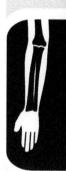

Practical – bony points and landmarks

You must be able to find on a model the following:

- Clavicle (whole length)
- Acromion
- Coracoid process
- Head of humerus
- Radial styloid
- Ulna shaft
- Posterior border of ulna
- Glenoid notch
- Spine of scapula
- Inferior angle scapula
- Greater tuberosity humerus
- Medial epicondyle humerus
- Lateral epicondyle humerus
- Radial head
- Olecranon
- Head of ulna
- Metacarpals 1–5
- All proximal phalanges
- All terminal phalanges
- Pisiform
- Scaphoid
- Hook of hamate

CHAPTER

Joints of the upper limb

Learning outcomes

After reading this chapter you should be able to:

1. Describe the structure of the joints of the upper limb including articular surfaces, movements possible, ligaments, capsule and other important features particular to that joint.

2. Describe the function of all joints of the upper limb.

3. Be able to relate 1 (above) to 2 (above).

4. Have a working knowledge of limiting factors to movements of the joints of the upper limb.

THE SHOULDER GIRDLE COMPLEX

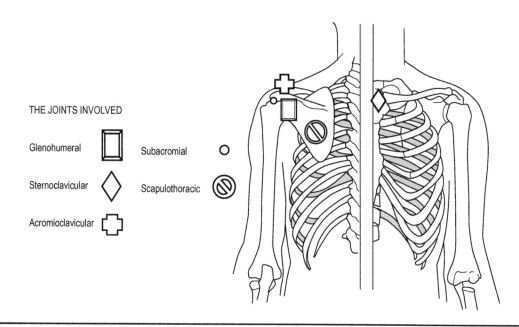

THE JOINTS INVOLVED

Glenohumeral □   Subacromial ○

Sternoclavicular ◇   Scapulothoracic ⊘

Acromioclavicular ✚

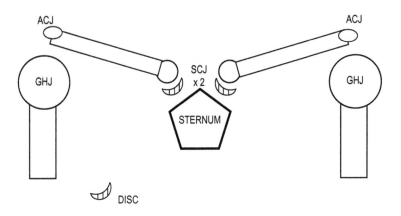

The plane of the scapula

As the wings of a *plane* sweep at an angle, so does the scapula as it sits on the thorax. Movements at the hip were described in pure anatomical planes. Well, just to make your student life a little more difficult this is not the case for the shoulder joint.

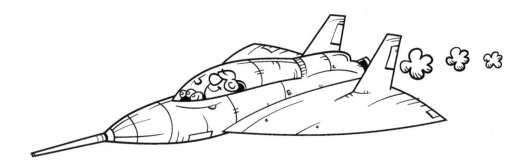

More on the plane of the scapula

Think back to what you learned about the hip joint. Remember how flexion was in the frontal plane, abduction was in a transverse plane and so on – the situation at the shoulder is not that simple. If you look at a person's scapulae, you will see that they lie posteriorly and also slightly protracted in the resting position. For this reason measurements of the shoulder joint are off-set slightly.

Professor asks

1. There is a joint between the humerus and the scapula called ....
2. There is a joint between sternum and clavicle called ....
3. There is a joint between acromion and clavicle called ....
4. What is the subacromial joint? ....
5. What is the scapulothoracic joint? ....

Answers
1. The glenohumeral joint.
2. The sternoclavicular joint.
3. The acromioclavicular joint.
4. The false joint formed underneath the acromion and including the subacromial bursa.
5. The term for the site where the scapula 'floats' on the thoracic wall.

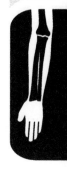

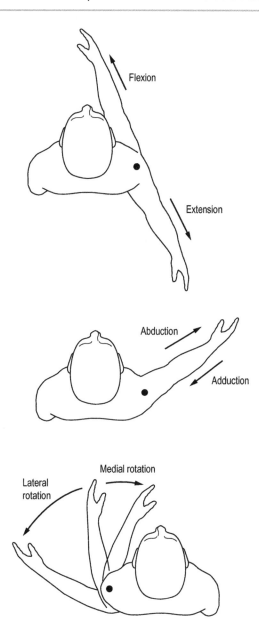

The sternoclavicular joint (SCJ)

Believe it or not, this is the only bony point of contact between the arm and the chest.

It is between the medial end of the clavicle and the superolateral angle of the sternum and 1st costal cartilage. The joint surfaces are not congruent – but this is minimised by the presence of an intra-articular disc.

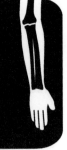

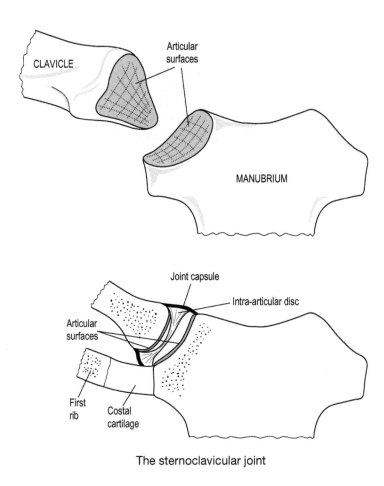

The sternoclavicular joint

The fibrous capsule of the SCJ

This is in the form of a sleeve around the joint. It is strong and is reinforced by anterior and posterior sternoclavicular ligaments and an interclavicular ligament.

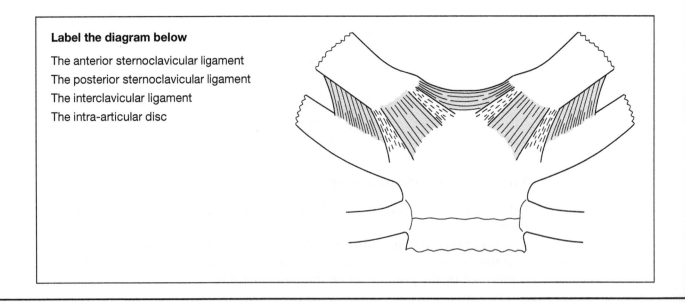

Label the diagram below

The anterior sternoclavicular ligament

The posterior sternoclavicular ligament

The interclavicular ligament

The intra-articular disc

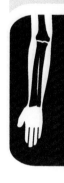

The SCJ is divided into two distinct cavities by the presence of a disc. The joint therefore has two synovial membranes! The disc:

☞ Improves joint congruency. What does this statement mean?
  Answer: It makes the bones fit together better.

Movements of the sternoclavicular joint

There are five degrees of freedom of motion:

☞ elevation
☞ depression
☞ protraction
☞ retraction
☞ axial rotation.

The axis for all these except axial rotation is the costoclavicular ligament.

Movements of the clavicle

Think of the clavicle as a see-saw, with the pivot being the costoclavicular ligament (cc below); as one end goes up, the other falls.

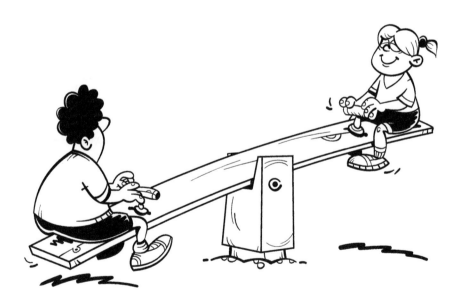

Make a more detailed study of the costoclavicular ligament, including clavicular movements and limiting factors to movements

The acromioclavicular joint (ACJ)

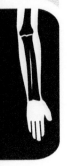

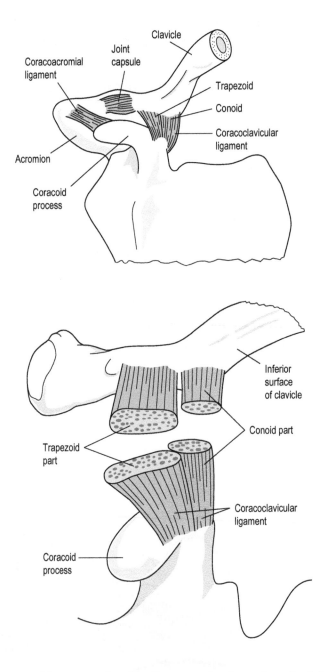

This joint is synovial between the flat facet on the lateral end of the clavicle and the flat facet on the anteromedial border of the acromion. Both surfaces are covered in fibrocartilage. Because of the shape and alignments of the surfaces, dislocations of the ACJ usually result in the acromion being displaced downwards and underneath the clavicle. The capsule is thickest above (superiorly) and is reinforced by trapezius. It is lined by synovial membrane. It usually possesses a wedge-shaped disc which increases joint congruency.

No muscles move the ACJ alone, none connect the two bones, but all movements of the scapula include movements of both (ACJ and SCJ).

The coracoclavicular ligament

Table 6.1 The coracoclavicular ligament

Conoid part	Trapezoid part
Attachments	Attachments
Structure	Structure
Function (limits forwards).	Function (limits backwards movement of the scapula)

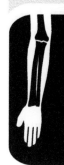

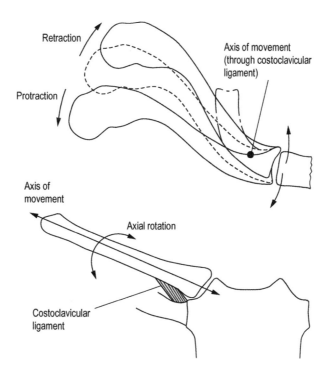

Remember the two parts of the coracoclavicular ligament (cc lig): Cutting corn requires a Con Traption (coracoid and trapezoid).

SCAPULAR ROTATION
The glenohumeral joint

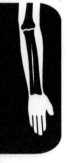

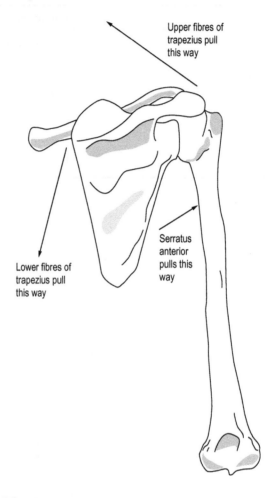

Upper fibres of
trapezius pull
this way

Lower fibres of
trapezius pull
this way

Serratus
anterior
pulls this
way

If you thought of the hip as an egg in an egg cup, think of the shoulder joint as a football resting on a saucer; the ball (humeral head) is too big for the saucer (glenoid) and the saucer is not really deep enough to stabilise the football.

So if the shoulder had to rely on the shape of its bones alone it would be very unstable. It needs help. It overcomes this problem by relying heavily on soft tissues which act as dynamic ligaments (the rotator cuff) rather like guy ropes on a tent.

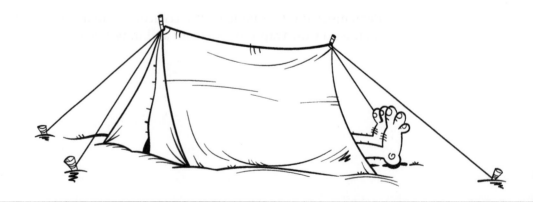

What does the shoulder joint do?

The function of the human shoulder is to place the hand in a functional position; hence it needs to be a very mobile joint but still keep a large amount of stability, fine movements, co-ordination, etc.

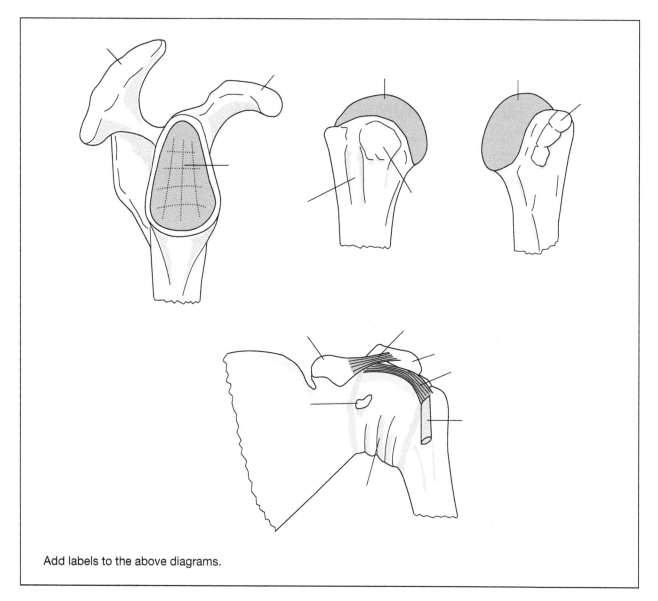
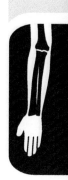

Add labels to the above diagrams.

Stop press: it *was* thought that the rotator cuff was the single most important factor in maintaining shoulder joint stability – it is now thought that also the negative pressure within the capsule helps cohesion of the bony surfaces. The biceps muscle also plays a role (see Chapter 7).

☞ Make sure that you fully understand the joints, bones and ligaments of the shoulder girdle. Can you discuss how these joints function in a living body?

☞ Why does the arrangement in the shoulder need to be different to that in the hip? Could you point out the structures of the shoulder girdle on
  – A model?
  – A skeleton?

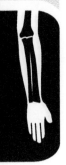

☞ Would you be able to talk about the shoulder girdle to:
- an examiner in your practical exams?
- a patient with *no* knowledge of anatomy?
- an orthopaedic surgeon?

☞ How would you modify your answers for each case above?

Stop press: the glenohumeral joint possesses a labrum rather like that found in the hip joint. It is increasingly being thought that problems with the labrum may be responsible for shoulder pain and instability (Jobe 1996).

SCAPULOHUMERAL RHYTHM

Abduction/elevation of the human shoulder girdle is complex. It is very import-ant that you understand this. Below is a simplified account of how it happens.

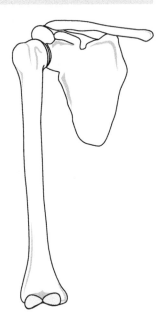

Starting point – arm by side.

Look up the latest biomechanical explanation for which muscles are active during this part of abduction.

Into more abduction, the scapula starts to rotate and tries to 'catch up' but never quite makes it. Force couple in action. Which muscles though? The greatest amount of relative scapular movement according to Bagg & Forrest (1988) is between 80 and 140° of arm abduction.

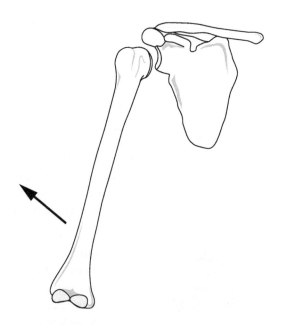

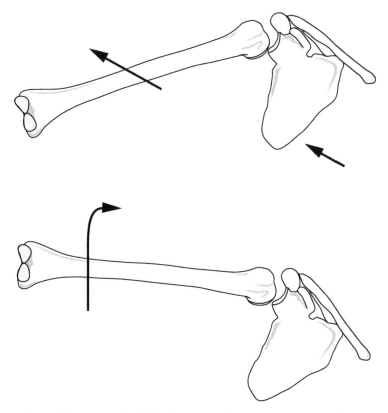

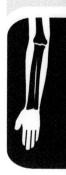

At approximately 90° of abduction, conjunct rotation of humerus has to happen to prevent the greater tuberosity of the humerus hitting the underside of the acromion.

The final few degrees of elevation is not by shoulder joint at all – it is done by scapular protraction = serratus anterior. If serratus anterior were weak what would you detect on examination?

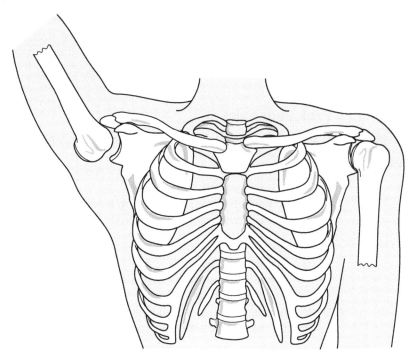

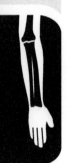

Professor says

Test yourself
Which muscles are represented by the three arrows on the scapula below?

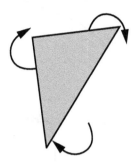

Answers

☞ Upper fibres of trapezius.
☞ Lower fibres of trapezius.
☞ Serratus anterior.

So what – why do I need to know?

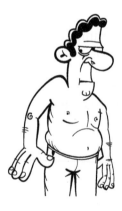

You need to understand a normal humeroscapular rhythm before you can spot an abnormal one – if a patient has rheumatoid arthritis affecting the shoulder, for example, the rotator cuff becomes severely degenerated and cannot perform its task of initiating abduction and stabilising the humeral head. The head of the humerus 'crashes' upwards into the underside of the acromion. Deltoid is left to cope and the patient will instead elevate the shoulder girdle first rather than as shown above. This makes the patient appear to hunch the shoulder – this is another important reason for you to expose the area when examining movements – it might appear that the man in the picture had 70° of abduction – he actually only has 20° at the glenohumeral joint!

Professor asks

1. If you had complete rupture of supraspinatus, which active movement would not be possible?
2. How might a patient manage to do the movement by 'cheating'? (sometimes known as a trick movement).
3. Why do patients sometimes develop a painful shoulder on the affected side following a CVA (cerebrovascular accident or stroke)?

Answers

1. Initiation of abduction.
2. They might lift the arm with the other arm or use a swinging movement to overcome the first few degrees of abduction.
3. Poor handling by people that overstretches soft tissues that have already lost tone and can result in instability and pain.

A STICKY PROBLEM

Look at how lax the glenohumeral capsule is inferiorly. This allows a huge range of movement at a normal glenohumeral joint.

These loose folds occasionally stick together, together with capsular contraction, severely restricting movements at the shoulder joint; this is a frozen shoulder – the correct term is adhesive capsulitis. A patient with this condition loses set proportions of movements – a capsular pattern.

You need to know the capsular patterns for the joints of the body.

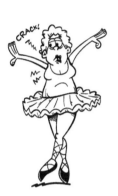

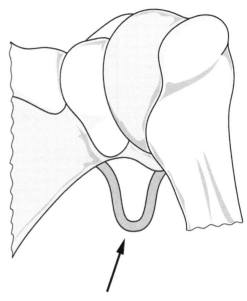

The capsule of the shoulder joint

HIP VERSUS SHOULDER JOINT

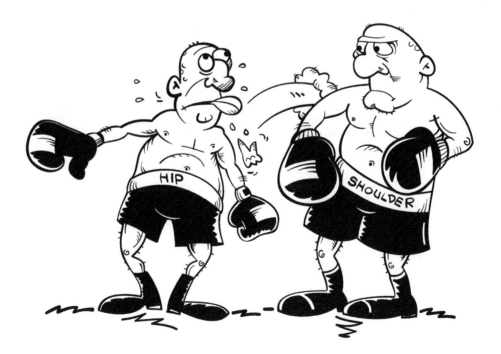

It might be useful for you to compare and contrast these two joints so that you can prove to yourself that your knowledge is increasing – or maybe not!

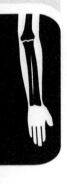

Complete this table:

Table 6.2

	Hip joint	Shoulder joint
Type of joint		
Degrees of freedom of movement		
Internal ligament		
Labrum		
Factors providing stability		
Factors allowing mobility		
Ease of dislocation		
Common direction of dislocation		
Major muscle groups		

GIVING YOU 'THE ELBOW' ⇐ A JOKE

The elbow is an important joint as once again its function is to place the hand in a useful position – ask anybody who has a fractured elbow how difficult it is to wash and eat!

Professor says

A fracture is the same as a break in medicine!

THE BONES OF THE ELBOW JOINT

☞ Distal humerus.
☞ Proximal radius.
☞ Proximal ulna.

The distal humerus has a trochlea and a capitulum.

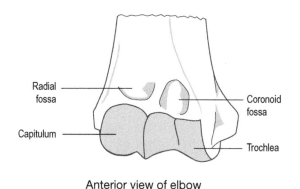

Radial
fossa

Capitulum

Coronoid
fossa

Trochlea

Anterior view of elbow

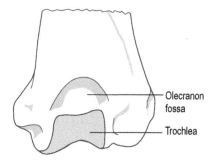

Olecranon
fossa

Trochlea

Posterior view of elbow

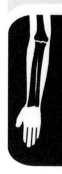

Using your classmates or friends, look at three male elbow joints and three female elbow joints

Do they differ? How do they differ? Why do they differ?

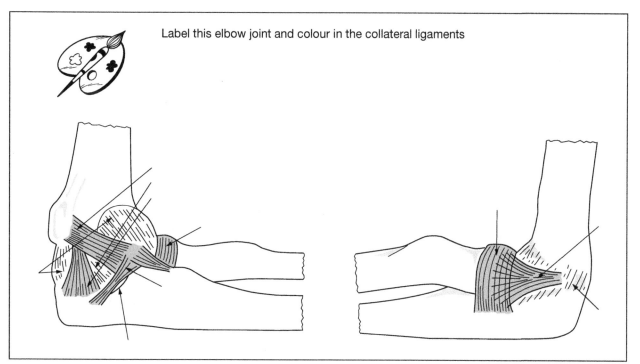

Label this elbow joint and colour in the collateral ligaments

The elbow has strong collateral ligaments – bunched at the sides of the joint so as not to interfere with the movements of flexion and extension. Look at an elbow from the side, the trochlea notch bulges anteriorly at an angle of 45°; this allows more flexion to occur. The ulna deviates 10–15° in males and 20–25° in females.

The elbow joint capsule

A capsule envelops the joint, from the medial epicondyle to the coronoid/radial fossae, posteriorly it follows the capitulum and arches upwards around the olecranon.

The elbow's collateral ligaments

These are strong triangular bands blended with the capsule. Like the knee they limit abduction and adduction. They are called the radial collateral and the ulnar collateral ligaments.

Palpation

Anteriorly muscles are in the way and the joint is not palpable. The joint line, however, is a line joining the two points, 1 cm below the lateral epicondyle and 2 cm below the medial epicondyle.

Stability

Stability comes from the elbow joint's bony shape; it is most stable in 90° of flexion (this is where most daily activities occur).

Movement

Movement of the elbow consists of flexion and extension, occurring through the carrying angle. Accessory movements of ab- and adduction are possible with the elbow in extension.

There is also a joint between the radius and ulna (superior radio-ulnar joint) and the radius and ulna also articulate with one another inferiorly (no prizes for guessing the name of this joint!).

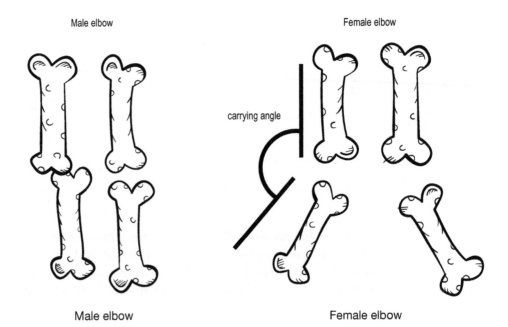

Male elbow

Female elbow

carrying angle

Male elbow

Female elbow

RADIO-ULNAR MOVEMENTS

Humero-ulnar joint	Radio-ulnar joint
Flexion Extension	Pronation Supination

RADIUS   ULNA

Limiting factors in the normal elbow joint

Flexion: soft tissue approximation.

Extension: bony block.

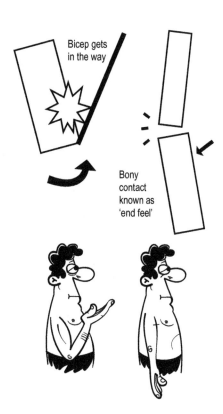

Bicep gets in the way

Bony contact known as 'end feel'

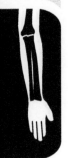

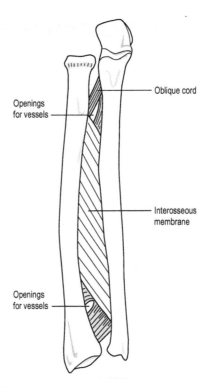

The radius and ulna articulated together

How to remember pronation and supination

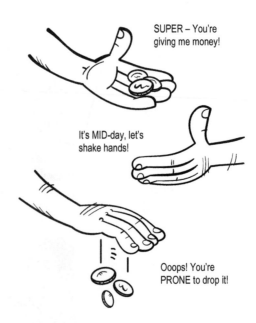

The annular ligament

The annular ligament grips the radial head like the cuff on a crutch.

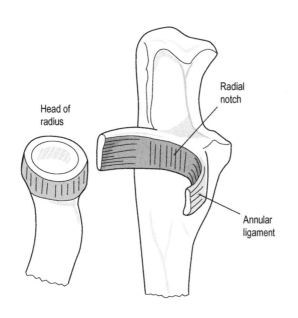

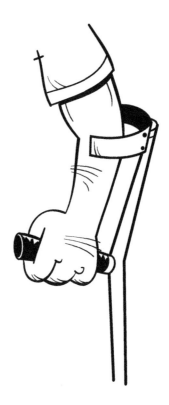

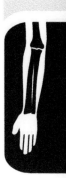

THE WRIST JOINT

The wrist is a complex joint and its function is closely linked with hand and radio-ulnar joint function. The wrist joint possesses an intra-articular disc. Arthroscopy of the wrist is now common and repairs to the disc complex can be performed using keyhole techniques (Cober & Trumble 2001).

The wrist possesses collateral ligaments and movements possible include flexion, extension, abduction and adduction.

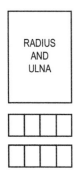

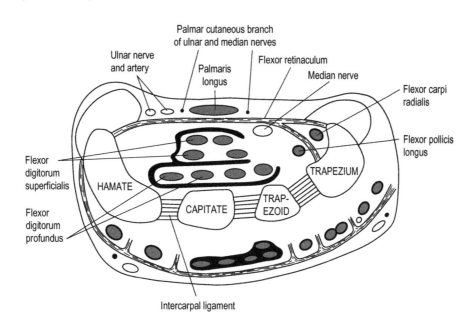

Transverse section through the wrist

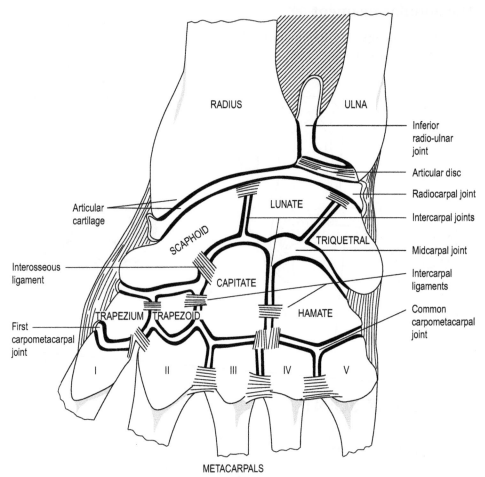

The carpus

Intercarpal joint

☞ Two rows of four bones.
☞ Minimal movement between bones.
☞ Dorsal, palmar, interosseous intercarpal ligaments present.

Midcarpal joint

☞ Between the two rows of carpal bones.
☞ Possesses dorsal, palmar, interosseous ligaments and incorporates radial and ulnar collateral ligaments.

Midcarpal movements

☞ Flexion – 50° possible.
☞ Extension – 35° possible.
☞ Abduction – 8° possible.
☞ Adduction – 15° possible.

Intermetacarpal joints

☞ Plane synovial.
☞ Palmar and dorsal ligaments.
☞ Small amplitude gliding movements occur here.

Carpometacarpal joint of the thumb

☞ Mobile but stable too (remember the hip joint?).
☞ Between trapezium and base of 1st metacarpal.
☞ The classic example of a saddle joint.

Professor says

Summarise the movements and limiting factors to movements of these joints.

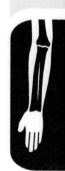

Metacarpophalangeal joints (MCP)

☞ Synovial condyloid joint.
☞ Two degrees of freedom of movement: flexion/extension and abduction/adduction.
☞ Some accessory rotation possible, in fact essential for normal movement, e.g. when gripping a ball.

Interphalangeal joints

On your own:

☞ Classify them.
☞ What are their main ligaments?
☞ Which movements are possible?

MOVEMENTS OF THE THUMB

Just to make life difficult for you the thumb does not lie in the same plane as the other fingers; as a result all measurements are different and can appear confusing at times. You need to understand the movement of the thumb, so I want you to add notes.

Complete this table.

Table 6.3

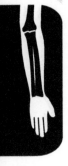

Movement	Definition	Muscles producing it	Functional example	Limiting factors
Thumb flexion				
Thumb extension				
Thumb adduction				
Thumb opposition				
Thumb abduction				

LIMITING FACTORS

Complete this table.

Table 6.4

Joint	Limiting factors (in the normal joint)
Shoulder	
Flexion	
Extension	
Abduction	
Adduction	
Internal rotation	
External rotation	
ACJ	
SCJ	

(continued)

Table 6.4 (*Continued*)

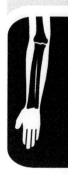

Joint	Limiting factors (in the normal joint)
Elbow	
Flexion	
Extension	
Superior radio-ulnar joint	
Pronation	
Supination	
Wrist joint	
Flexion	
Extension	
Abduction	
Adduction	
Metacarpophalangeal joints	
Flexion	
Extension	
Abduction	
Adduction	
Interphalangeal joints	
Flexion	
Extension	

How can I remember what passes through the carpal tunnel?

The carpal tunnel is like the M25 on a bad day, a busy place and not much room for mistakes.

Think of
4 **pro**fessors   = 4 **prof**undus tendons
on 4 scooters   = 4 **super**ficialis tendons
Nearby is a **fairly polite lady** = FPL tendon
with **mo**ney   = **m**edian nerve.

Judgement time

Before your written and practical examinations, go through each of these points; can you write about each in detail and demonstrate it practically?

You should be able to identify practically on a model and write about in detail for written exams:

Shoulder (glenohumeral)

- ❏ Joint line
- ❏ Movements
- ❏ Limiting factors to movement
- ❏ Bones involved
- ❏ Classification

Acromioclavicular and sternoclavicular

- ❏ Joint line
- ❏ Movements
- ❏ Limiting factors to movement
- ❏ Bones involved
- ❏ Classification
- ❏ Main ligaments

Elbow joint

- ❏ Palpate location
- ❏ Joint line
- ❏ Classification
- ❏ Ligaments
- ❏ Limiting factors to movement

Superior radio-ulnar joint

- ❏ Joint line
- ❏ Movements
- ❏ Limiting factors to movement
- ❏ Bones involved

- ❏ Classification
- ❏ Three lateral ligaments
- ❏ Medial (deltoid) ligament

Inferior radio-ulnar joint

- ❏ Movements
- ❏ Limiting factors to movement
- ❏ Bones involved
- ❏ Classification
- ❏ Ligaments

Wrist joint

- ❏ Bones involved
- ❏ Classification
- ❏ Movements possible
- ❏ Main ligaments

Midcarpal joint

- ❏ Bones involved
- ❏ Classification
- ❏ Movements possible
- ❏ Main ligaments

Metacarpophalangeal and interphalangeal joints

- ❏ Bones involved
- ❏ Classification
- ❏ Movements possible
- ❏ Main ligaments

7

Muscles of the upper limb

Learning outcomes

After reading this chapter, for each of the muscles you should be able to describe:

1. Origin.

2. Insertion.

3. Nerve supply.

MUSCLES AROUND THE SHOULDER GIRDLE

The muscles of the shoulder girdle are of the following types:

☞ Elevators and Depressors
☞ Protractors and Retractors
☞ Lateral rotators and Medial rotators.

Don't forget that muscles do many different things and these tables list their main actions only, so for example whilst biceps brachii is a flexor of the elbow, it is also a powerful supinator and the long head also flexes the shoulder joint.

Table 7.1

Muscle	Origin	Insertion	Action	Nerve supply
Levator scapulae	transverse processes of C1–C4 vertebrae	medial border of the scapula from the superior angle to the spine	elevates the scapula	dorsal scapular nerve (C5); the upper part of the muscle receives branches of C3 and C4
Trapezius	medial third of the superior nuchal line, external occipital protuberance, ligamentum nuchae, spinous processes of vertebrae C7–T12	lateral third of the clavicle, medial side of the acromion and the upper crest of the scapular spine, tubercle of the scapular spine	elevates (upper fibres) and depresses (lower fibres) the scapula; retracts the scapula	motor: spinal accessory (XI), proprioception: C3–C4

Table 7.2 Shoulder girdle retractors and protractors

Muscle	Origin	Insertion	Action	Nerve supply
Rhomboid major	spines of vertebrae T2–T5	medial border of the scapula inferior to the spine of the scapula	retracts, elevates and rotates the scapula inferiorly	dorsal scapular nerve (C5)
Rhomboid minor	inferior end of the ligamentum nuchae, spines of vertebrae C7 and T1	medial border of the scapula at the root of the spine of the scapula	retracts, elevates and rotates the scapula inferiorly	dorsal scapular nerve (C5)
Serratus anterior	ribs 1–8 or 9	medial border of the scapula on its costal (deep) surface	it draws the scapula forward; the inferior fibres rotate the scapula superiorly	long thoracic nerve (from ventral rami C5–C7)
Pectoralis major	medial half of the clavicle, manubrium and body of sternum, costal cartilages of ribs 2–6	greater tubercle of the humerus	flexes and adducts the arm, medially rotates the arm	medial and lateral pectoral nerves (C5–T1)
Pectoralis minor	ribs 3–5	coracoid process of the scapula	draws the scapula forward, medialward, and downward	medial pectoral nerve (C8, T1)

Ask a model (topless!) to push against a wall with their elbows extended. Stand behind them and observe their scapulae. Serratus anterior works hard to prevent their nose hitting the wall – it is a similar movement to doing a 'press up'. If serratus anterior is weak, a 'winged scapula' results. This means that the scapula is not held against the thorax as it should be and 'sticks out' especially the medial border and inferior angle.

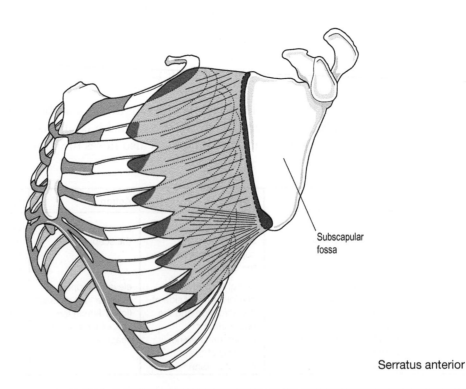

Subscapular fossa

Serratus anterior

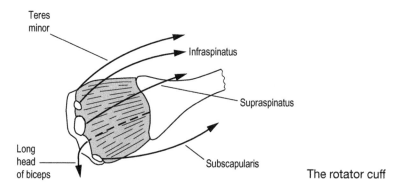

The rotator cuff

Table 7.3   The rotator cuff is very important – you should know it in detail. Here are its components

Muscle	Origin	Insertion	Action	Nerve supply
Subscapularis	medial two-thirds of the costal surface of the scapula (subscapular fossa)	lesser tubercle of the humerus	medially rotates the arm	upper and lower subscapular nerves
Supraspinatus	supraspinatous fossa	greater tubercle of the humerus (highest facet)	abducts the arm (initiates abduction)	suprascapular nerve (C5,6) from the superior trunk of brachial plexus
Infraspinatus	infraspinatous fossa	greater tubercle of the humerus (middle facet)	laterally rotates the arm	suprascapular nerve
Teres minor	upper two-thirds of the lateral border of the scapula	greater tubercle of the humerus (lowest facet)	laterally rotates the arm	axillary nerve (C5,6) from the posterior cord of the brachial plexus

Professor asks

If the rotator cuff is so fabulous, then why is there not a rotator cuff in the hip joint?

Answer

It doesn't need one – the hip is less reliant on soft tissues for its stability than the shoulder.

An easy way to remember the relative positions of the rotator cuff muscles.

Remember: **SubSIT**.

Starting from the most anterior, this tells you their positions:

☞ **Sub** (scapularis)
☞ **S** (upraspinatus)
☞ **I** (nfraspinatus)
☞ **T** (eres minor)

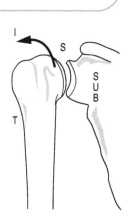

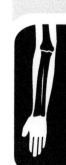

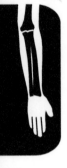

Supraspinatus

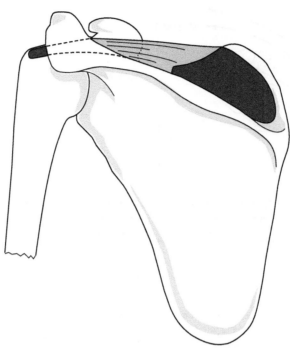

Questions
1. What does 'supra' mean?
2. What does 'spinatus' mean?
3. Which other muscles make up the rotator cuff?
4. What is the action of the rotator cuff?
5. Supraspinatus lesions frequently exhibit a painful arc – what is this?

Answers
1. Above.
2. The spine (of scapula).
3. Infraspinatus teres minor subscapularis.
4. Acts as a set of dynamic ligaments controlling the position of the humeral head.
5. Pain felt in middle range abduction – consult a soft tissue injuries text.

More 'off the cuff' comments

One of the most important functions of the rotator cuff is to surround and support the humeral head. If I gave you a bundle of money (yeah right!) that you wanted to hold securely, you would grab it, wrapping your fingers around the money so that from all directions the money would be secure.

Think of the rotator cuff in this way, surrounding the head of the humerus to give the shoulder stability, yet adaptable enough to allow a large number of fine movements. A person who has suffered a stroke (cerebrovascular incident) may lose muscle tone in their rotator cuff – hence the shoulder becomes unstable and subluxes; it is quite common to find painful shoulders in these patients. Now you know why.

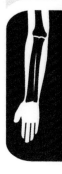

Stop press: one of the newer theories about how the shoulder joint maintains its stability focuses on the negative pressure within the joint – a bit like sucking the air out of a balloon, the edges of the balloon are held together. Bearing this in mind, why do some surgeons now believe that arthroscopy of the shoulder causes problems in itself?

A friend comes to see you, he has been diagnosed as having a torn rotator cuff. Nobody has explained this to him and he is very worried about what this means exactly – write down what you would say to him. If you wish, show the finished product to a lecturer for their comments; better still, show it to a friend who knows nothing about anatomy – see if they understand it. It is one thing being able to write wonderful essays but no use to you if you cannot get the information across simply and in a form that is understood by non-health care professionals.

Deltoid

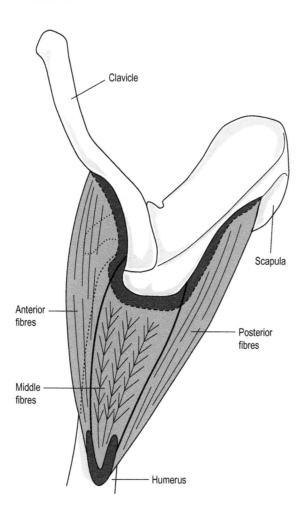

1. The middle fibres of deltoid are multipennate, what does this statement mean?
2. The anterior fibres of deltoid lie anterior to the glenohumeral joint therefore they will assist with .... of the shoulder.

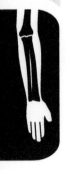

3. The posterior fibres of deltoid lie posterior to the glenohumeral joint therefore they will assist with .... of the shoulder.
4. Which muscle assists deltoid by initiating abduction of the shoulder?

Answers
1. Look it up in Chapter 1 under morphology of muscle.
2. Flexion.
3. Extension.
4. Supraspinatus.

Latissimus dorsi

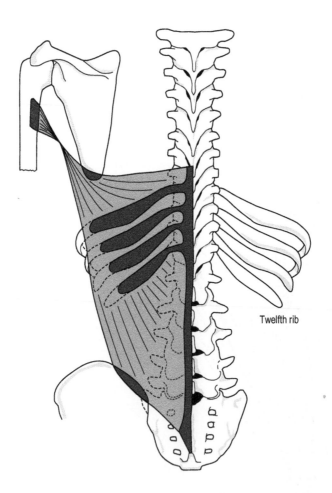

Twelfth rib

This huge muscle gives bodybuilders their V shape. It has attachments as low as the ilium, so it can achieve hitching of the pelvis if its action is reversed (insertion remains fixed and origin moves instead).

Trapezius

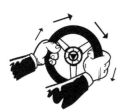

A = direction of pull of upper trapezius fibres
B = direction of pull of lower trapezius fibres
C = direction of pull of serratus anterior

The combined result of this force couple is scapular rotation, rather like steering a car by using two opposite movements on either side of the wheel.

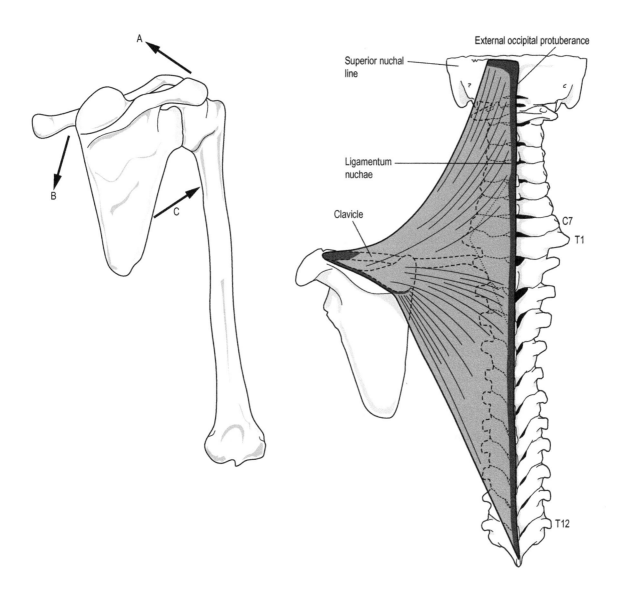

Table 7.4

Muscle	Origin	Insertion	Action	Nerve supply
Pectoralis major	medial half of the clavicle; manubrium and body of sternum; costal cartilages of ribs 2–6; sometimes from the rectus sheath of the upper abdominal wall	crest of the greater tubercle of the humerus	flexes and adducts the arm; medially rotates the arm	medial and lateral pectoral nerves (C5–T1)
Deltoid	lateral one-third of the clavicle; acromion; lower lip of the crest of the spine of the scapula	deltoid tuberosity of the humerus	abducts the arm; anterior fibres flex and medially rotate the humerus; posterior fibres extend and laterally rotate the humerus	axillary nerve (C5,6) from the posterior cord of the brachial plexus
Biceps brachii	short head: tip of the coracoid process of the scapula; long head: supraglenoid tubercle of the scapula	tuberosity of the radius	flexes the elbow (long head flexes shoulder); supinates	musculocutaneous nerve (C5,6)
Brachioradialis, superior aspect of styloid process of radius	upper lateral supracondylar ridge of humerus; lateral intermuscular septum of humerus	lateral side of the distal half to one-third of the radius	flexes the forearm at the elbow; pronates the forearm when supinated; supinates the forearm when pronated	radial nerve, C5,6

Table 7.5 Shoulder extensors

Muscle	Origin	Insertion	Action	Nerve supply
Latissimus dorsi	vertebral spines from T7 to the sacrum; posterior third of the iliac crest; lower three or four ribs; sometimes from the inferior angle of the scapula	floor of the inter-tubercular groove	extends and medially rotates the shoulder	thoracodorsal nerve (C7,8) from the posterior cord of the brachial plexus
Teres major	dorsal surface of the inferior angle of the scapula	crest of the lesser tubercle of the humerus	adducts the shoulder, medially rotates the arm, assists in arm extension	lower subscapular nerve (C5,6) from the posterior cord of the brachial plexus

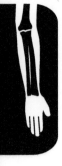

Shoulder extensors

Biceps brachii – two heads are better than one. And the jokes just keep on coming!

☞ What does the word biceps mean?
☞ What does brachii mean?
☞ What does biceps do:
    (a) at the glenohumeral joint?
    (b) at the elbow joint?
    (c) at the radio-ulnar joint?
☞ What signs and symptoms would you expect following a rupture (complete snapping) of the long head of biceps?

Answers

☞ Two heads.

☞ Arm.

☞ (a) Flexes the elbow joint; (b) flexion at the glenohumeral joint (via its long head); (c) supinates the forearm.

☞ Sudden snap may be felt. Shoulder pain (or not). Arm will take on appearance of Popeye muscle as muscle belly shunts distally.

On this diagram label the long and short heads and the bicipital aponeurosis of the biceps brachii.

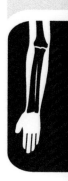

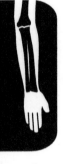

Andrews *et al.* (1985) made these observations about biceps:
   'Only the biceps brachii traverses both the elbow joint and the shoulder joint. Additional forces are generated in the biceps tendon in its function as a shunt muscle to stabilise the glenohumeral joint during the throwing act.'

Professor says

'Let's hear it for the left handers!'

Supination is more powerful than pronation so left-handed people are better at removing screws that are stubborn!

Remember a symptom is what a person complains of, a sign is what can be measured or tested for

ELBOW FLEXORS

Table 7.6

Muscle	Origin	Insertion	Nerve supply
Biceps brachii	long head: supraglenoid tubercle and glenohumeral labrum; short head: tip of the coracoid	radial tuberosity; bicipital aponeurosis	musculocutaneous nerve, C5,6
Brachialis	lower half of anterior humerus	ulnar tuberosity; coronoid process of ulna	musculocutaneous nerve, C5,6
Coracobrachialis	coracoid process	medial shaft of the humerus	musculocutaneous nerve, C5,6,(C7)

ELBOW EXTENSORS

Table 7.7

Muscle	Origin	Insertion	Nerve supply
Triceps brachii	long head: infraglenoid tubercle of scapula; lateral head: upper portion of posterior surface of the shaft of the humerus; medial head: posterior shaft of humerus, distal to radial groove and both the medial and lateral intermuscular septum (deep to the long and lateral heads)	posterior surface of the olecranon process of the ulna	radial nerve, C6,7
Anconeus	posterior surface of the lateral epicondyle of the humerus	lateral aspect of olecranon	radial nerve, C7,8

Triceps

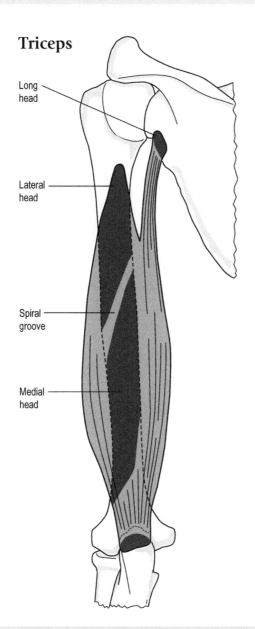

Long head

Lateral head

Spiral groove

Medial head

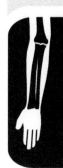

PRONATION AND SUPINATION

Table 7.8

Muscle	Origin	Insertion	Nerve supply
Pronator teres	humeral head: upper portion of medial epicondyle, medial brachial intermuscular septum; ulnar head: coronoid process of ulna	lateral aspect of radius at the middle of the shaft (pronator tuberosity)	median nerve, C6,7
Pronator quadratus	distal quarter anteromedial surface of ulna	distal quarter anterolateral surface of radius	anterior interosseous branch of median nerve, C8,T1
Supinator	lateral epicondyle of humerus, supinator crest of ulna, radial collateral ligament, annular ligament	proximal portion of anterolateral surface of the radius	deep branch of the radial nerve, C6

FLEXION AT THE WRIST JOINT

Table 7.9

Muscle	Origin	Insertion	Nerve supply
Flexor carpi radialis	medial epicondyle via the CFT (common flexor tendon)	base of the second and sometimes third metacarpals	median nerve, C6,7
Palmaris longus	medial epicondyle via the CFT (common flexor tendon)	central portion of the flexor retinaculum; superficial portion of the palmar aponeurosis	median nerve, C6,7
Flexor carpi ulnaris	humeral head: medial epicondyle via the CFT (common flexor tendon); ulnar head: medial aspect of olecranon and proximal three-fifths of dorsal ulnar shaft	pisiform and hamate bones (via the pisohamate ligament); base of the 5th metacarpal (via the pisometacarpal ligament)	ulnar nerve, C8,T1

What a load of pollux!

The word **Pollicis** = thumb; the word **hallux** = toe.

How to remember the finger flexor tendons and their arrangement

It can be **profound**ly difficult to thread unless you have a **super** needle (**profundus** threads through **super**ficialis tendon).

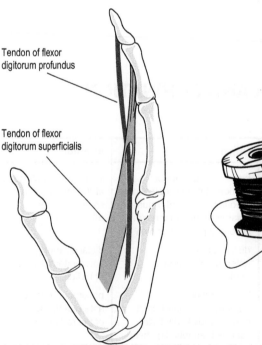

Tendon of flexor digitorum profundus

Tendon of flexor digitorum superficialis

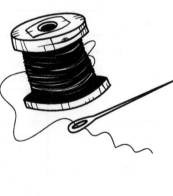

EXTENSION AT THE WRIST JOINT

Table 7.10

Muscle	Origin	Insertion	Action	Nerve supply
Extensor carpi radialis longus	lower lateral supracondylar ridge (below the brachio-radialis); lateral intermuscular septum of humerus	base of second metacarpal	extends the hand at the wrist; radially deviates the hand at the wrist; weakly flexes the forearm; weakly supinates	radial nerve, C5,6
Extensor carpi radialis brevis	lateral epicondyle via the CET (common extensor tendon); radial collateral ligament	base of third metacarpal	extends the wrist; radially deviates the hand	radial nerve, C6,7
Extensor digitorum	lateral epicondyle via the CET (common extensor tendon)	base of middle phalanx of each of the four fingers (central band); base of distal phalanx of each of the four fingers (two lateral bands)	extends four medial digits; extends the wrist if fingers are flexed; abducts the digits	posterior interosseous nerve of the radial nerve, C6,7,8
Extensor digiti minimi	lateral epicondyle via the CET (common extensor tendon); antebrachial fascia; ulnar aspect of extensor digitorum	base of middle phalanx of the fifth digit (central band); base of distal phalanx of the fifth digit (two lateral bands)	extends fifth digit; abducts fifth digit	posterior interosseous nerve of the radial nerve, C6,7,8
Extensor carpi ulnaris	first head: lateral epicondyle via the CET (common extensor tendon); second head: posterior body of ulna, antebrachial fascia	medial side of base of the fifth metacarpal	extends the hand at the wrist; ulnarly deviates the hand at the wrist	posterior interosseous nerve of the radial nerve, C6,7,8

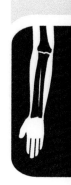

FLEXION OF THE FINGERS/THUMB

Table 7.11

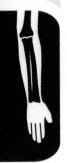

Muscle	Origin	Insertion	Action	Nerve supply
Flexor digitorum superficialis	humeral-ulnar head: medial epicondyle via the CFT (common flexor tendon), medial border of base of coronoid process of ulna, medial (ulnar) collateral ligament; radial head: oblique line of radius	both sides of the base of each middle phalanx of the four fingers	flexes the proximal and middle phalanges; flexes the wrist if fingers are extended	median nerve, C7,8,T1
Flexor digitorum profundus	anterior and medial surface of upper three-quarters of ulna; adjacent interosseous membrane	insertion: distal phalanx of medial four digits (through FDS tunnel)	flexes the distal IP joints and in so doing flexes the proximal and middle IP joints; flexes the wrist if fingers are extended	medial portion: ulnar nerve, C8,T1; lateral portion: anterior interosseous branch of median nerve, C8,T1
Lumbricals	tendon of flexor digitorum profundus; 1 & 2 have a single head of origin (from radial aspect of tendon); 3 & 4 have two heads of origin (each head from an adjacent tendon)	extensor hood of digits 2–5	flexes the fingers (at the MCP joints); extend IPs	1 & 2: median nerve, C8,T1; 3 & 4: deep branch of ulnar nerve, C8,T1
Flexor digiti minimi brevis	distal border of flexor retinaculum; hook of the hamate	medial aspect of the base of proximal phalanx	flexes the fifth digit (at the MCP joint)	deep branch of ulnar nerve, C8,T1
Flexor pollicis longus	middle anterior surface of the radius; interosseous membrane	insertion: palmar aspect of base of the distal phalanx of thumb	flexes the distal phalanx of the thumb (IP joint); flexes the other joints to the wrist (MCP, CMC and weakly at the wrist)	Anterior interosseous branch of median nerve, C8,T1
Flexor pollicis brevis	superficial head: distal border of flexor retinaculum; trapezium; deep head: floor of carpal tunnel indirectly to scaphoid and trapezium	base of proximal phalanx of thumb; can also attach to the lateral sesamoid bone at the MCP joint	Action: powerfully flexes the thumb (at the MCP joint)	superficial head: recurrent branch of median nerve, C8,T1; deep head: deep branch of ulnar nerve, C8,T1

EXTENSION OF THE FINGERS/THUMB

Table 7.12

Muscle	Origin	Insertion	Action	Nerve supply
Extensor digitorum	lateral epicondyle via the CET (common extensor tendon)	base of middle phalanx of each of the four fingers (central band); base of distal phalanx of each of the four fingers (two lateral bands)	extends the four medial digits; extends the wrist if fingers flexed; abducts the digits (spreads the digits as it extends them)	posterior interosseous nerve of the radial nerve, C6,7,8
Extensor digiti minimi	lateral epicondyle via the CET (common extensor tendon)	base of middle phalanx of the fifth digit (central band); base of distal phalanx of the fifth digit (two lateral bands)	extends the fifth digit; abducts the fifth digit	posterior interosseous nerve of the radial nerve, C6,7,8
Extensor indicis	posterior surface of ulna (distal to extensor pollicis longus); interosseous membrane	base of middle and distal phalanx of the index finger	extends the second digit (MCP and IP joints); adducts the second digit; assists to extend the hand at the wrist; stabilises MCP joint for flexion of IP solely	posterior interosseous nerve of the radial nerve, C6,7,8

ABDUCTION/ADDUCTION/OPPOSITION OF THE FINGERS

Table 7.13

Muscle	Origin	Insertion	Action	Nerve supply
Palmar interossei	from the side of the metacarpal that faces the mid-line – to adduct them	on the base of the proximal phalanx of the digit of origin (same side toward the mid-line); extensor hood of the same digit(s)	adducts the fingers (hint: PAD = Palmar ADduct); flexes the fingers (at the MCP while IP joints are extended)	deep branch of ulnar nerve, C8,T1
Dorsal interossei	between each metacarpal	directly distal to the origin on the base of the proximal phalanx closest to the mid-line (to abduct them); extensor hood of the same digit(s)	abducts the fingers (hint: DAB = Dorsal ABduct); flexes the fingers (at the MCP while IP joints are extended)	deep branch of ulnar nerve, C8,T1
Palmaris brevis	palmar aponeurosis	skin of ulnar border of palm	tenses the skin on the ulnar side, which is used in a grip action	superficial branch of ulnar nerve, C8,T1
Abductor digiti minimi	pisiform and tendon of flexor carpi ulnaris	medial aspect of the base of proximal phalanx of the fifth digit	abduct fifth digit (requires pisiform stabilised by FCU); assists to flex the fifth digit (at MCP); may assist in extension of fifth digit (at IP due to slips to extensor digitorum)	deep branch of ulnar nerve, C8,T1
Opponens digiti minimi	distal border of flexor retinaculum; hook of the hamate	medial aspect of the fifth metacarpal	opposes the fifth digit with the thumb; assists to 'cup' the palm	deep branch of ulnar nerve, C8,T1

MUSCLES ACTING ON THE THUMB

Table 7.14

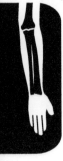

Muscle	Origin	Insertion	Action	Nerve supply
Abductor pollicis	posterior surfaces of ulna and radius; interosseous membrane	lateral aspect of base of first metacarpal	abducts the first metacarpal; assists to extend and rotate the thumb; radially deviates the hand at the wrist; flexes the hand at the wrist	posterior interosseous nerve of the radial nerve, C6,7,(C8)
Extensor pollicis brevis	posterior surfaces of radius (below abductor pollicis longus); interosseous membrane	base of proximal phalanx of thumb (often a slip inserts into extensor pollicis longus tendon)	extends the proximal phalanx and first metacarpal of the thumb; radially deviates the hand at the wrist	posterior interosseous nerve of the radial nerve, C6,7,(C8)
Extensor pollicis longus	posterior surface of ulna; interosseous membrane	distal phalanx of thumb	extends distal phalanx of thumb; extends proximal phalanx of thumb; assists to extend the hand at the wrist (if fingers flexed)	posterior interosseous nerve of the radial nerve, C6,7,8
Abductor pollicis brevis	distal border of flexor retinaculum	lateral aspect of base of proximal phalanx of the thumb; may also send a slip to the tendon of extensor pollicis longus	abducts thumb (at the MCP joint); participates to flex the thumb (at the MCP joint)	median nerve, C8,T1
Opponens pollicis	distal border of flexor retinaculum; trapezium	lateral aspect of the first metacarpal	opposes the thumb to the fingers	recurrent branch of median nerve, C8,T1
Adductor pollicis tunnel	transverse head: third metacarpal; oblique head: base of first, second and third metacarpals; floor of carpal tunnel	medial aspect of the base of proximal phalanx; medial sesamoid at MCP	adducts the thumb; may assist to flex the thumb (at the MCP joint)	deep branch of ulnar nerve, C8,T1

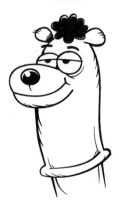

Meet 'Larry the Lumbrical'

The lumbricals flex the MCP joints and extend the PIPs rather like the position you would place your hand in when making a 'Larry the Lumbrical' glove puppet.
(Larry the Lumbrical was thought up by Claire Cooper – with thanks.)

Judgement time

For all muscles of the upper limb you need to know:

- ❏ Origin
- ❏ Insertion
- ❏ Nerve supply.

1. Write individual muscles' names on separate cards, randomly pick cards and make sure that you can describe origin, action, insertion and nerve supply for the muscle chosen.
2. For each muscle in the upper limb, think of a functional activity for which that muscle might be needed.
3. While you are watching your favourite TV programme analyse the muscle activity you can see in the living body.

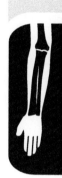

CHAPTER

Nerves of the upper limb

Learning outcomes

After reading this chapter you should be able to describe

1. Root level.
2. Relations.
3. Major branches.
4. Innervations of the
   - Musculocutaneous nerve
   - Axillary nerve

- Median nerve
- Ulnar nerve
- Radial nerve.

You need to know the dermatomes and myotomes of the lower and upper limbs.

THE BRACHIAL PLEXUS

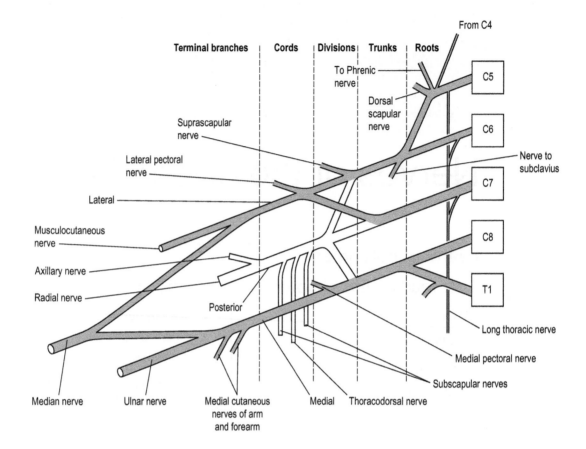

What is a plexus? A plexus is a network or tangle of nerves or veins.

How can I remember the divisions of the plexus?

Really	*Roots*
Tight	*Trunks*
Denims	*Divisions*
Cause	*Cords*
Blotches	*Branches*

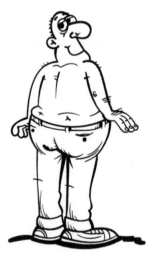

THE MUSCULOCUTANEOUS NERVE

(The BBC nerve!)

- ☞ Arises from lateral cord of brachial plexus C5, 6, 7.
- ☞ Descends between axillary artery and coracobrachialis, which it pierces.
- ☞ Then runs between biceps and coracobrachialis to reach lateral side of the arm.
- ☞ Pierces deep fascia at the elbow as the lateral cutaneous nerve of the arm.

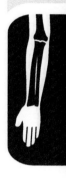

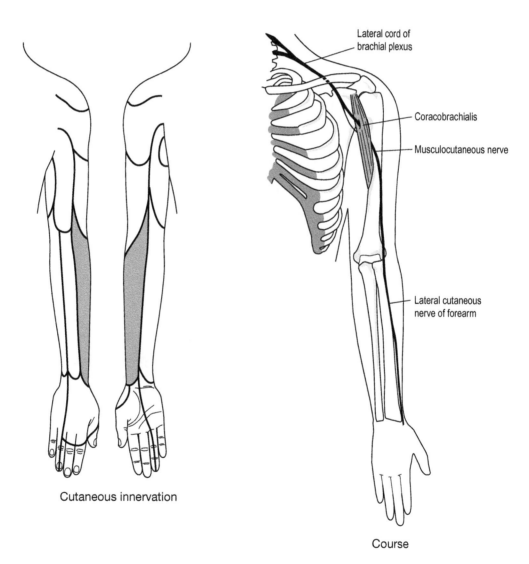

Cutaneous innervation

Course

The musculocutaneous nerve supplies Biceps, Brachialis and Coracobrachialis (remember BBC!).

THE AXILLARY NERVE

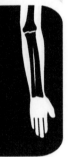

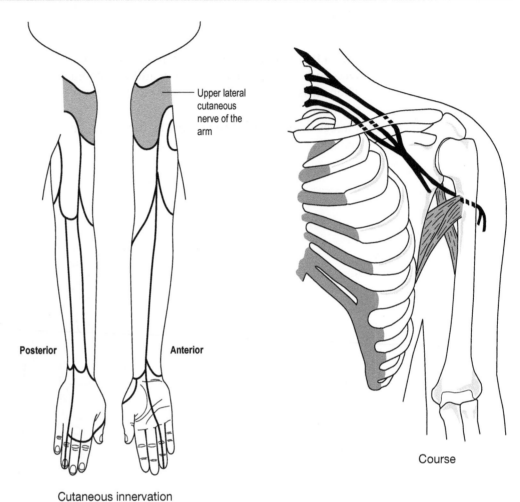

Upper lateral
cutaneous
nerve of the
arm

Posterior   Anterior

Course

Cutaneous innervation

☞ Arises from posterior cord brachial plexus C5, 6.
☞ Descends behind axillary artery in front of subscapularis.
☞ Passes inferior to shoulder joint then through quadrangular space.
☞ Supplies shoulder joint.
☞ Splits into anterior and posterior branches.
☞ Anterior branch winds round surgical neck of humerus to supply anterior deltoid.
☞ Posteriorly is teres minor, posterior fibres are deltoid and it continues as lateral cutaneous nerve of the arm – supplies skin over lower deltoid and lateral triceps.

The axillary nerve may be injured in shoulder dislocations – which muscles would be paralysed if this were the case?

THE MEDIAN NERVE

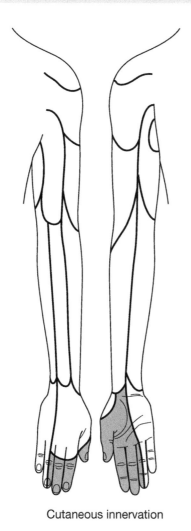

Cutaneous innervation

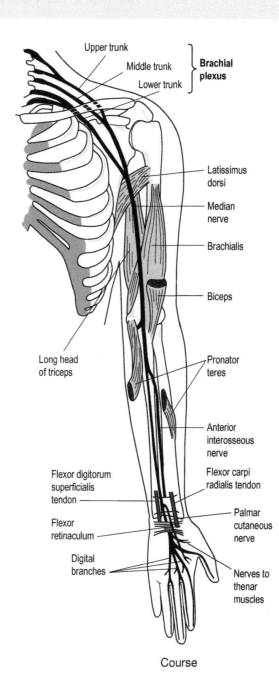

Course

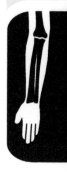

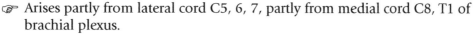

- ☞ Arises partly from lateral cord C5, 6, 7, partly from medial cord C8, T1 of brachial plexus.
- ☞ Descends under biceps lateral to brachial artery then medially.
- ☞ It lies on top of brachialis.
- ☞ Then is crossed by the bicipital aponeurosis.
- ☞ Enters the forearm between two heads of pronator teres.
- ☞ Travels between flexor digitorum profundus and superficialis.
- ☞ Becomes superficial at the wrist but deep to palmaris longus.
- ☞ Passes through the carpal tunnel.

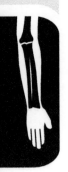

The median nerve sends articular branches to the elbow joint and supplies:

☞ pronator teres.
☞ flexor carpi radialis.
☞ palmaris longus.
☞ flexor digitorum superficialis.
☞ flexor digitorum profundus.
☞ flexor pollicis longus.
☞ pronator quadratus.

Once through the carpal tunnel, the median nerve enters the hand and it divides into lateral and medial branches. The lateral branch supplies abductor pollicis brevis, flexor pollicis brevis, opponens pollicis and first lumbrical. The medial branch supplies the second lumbrical, and has many digital branches to nail beds, IP joints and MCP joints.

The median nerve may be injured by deep cuts. This gives loss of flexion of IP joints, except for the distal ones in ring and little fingers. MCPs can still be flexed by lumbricals and interossei. Thumb cannot oppose or abduct deformity (monkey hand). The thumb lies in same plane as hand, with wasting of the thenar eminence.

Compression in the carpal tunnel or carpal tunnel syndrome affects the thenar muscles, lateral two lumbricals, and leads to sensory changes in the hand.

What can cause carpal tunnel syndrome?

THE RADIAL NERVE

☞ Posterior cord brachial plexus C5, 6, 7, 8 (T1).
☞ Passes anterior to subscapularis, latissimus dorsi and teres major.
☞ Enters spiral groove of humerus.
☞ Pierces intermuscular septum to enter anterior compartment to lie between brachialis and brachioradialis.
☞ In front of lateral humeral epicondyle, it splits into superficial and deep branches.

The radial nerve supplies mainly:

☞ triceps, anconeus
☞ brachioradialis
☞ ECRL, ECRB
☞ supinator
☞ long finger extensors
☞ abductor pollicis longus
☞ thumb extensors.

Injury to the radial nerve leads to an inability to extend wrist/fingers, with wrist drop. There is a loss of synergistic action of wrist extensors when making a fist (what does this statement mean?).

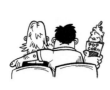

The radial nerve may be damaged by fracture to the humeral shaft where it winds round the bone – always check these fractures for signs of a wrist drop. It may be injured by axillary crutches used incorrectly.

What is a Saturday night palsy?

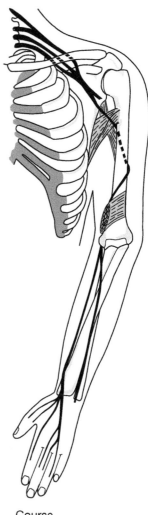

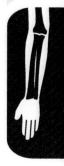

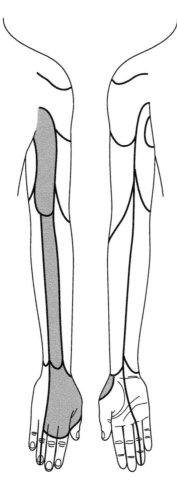

Cutaneous innervation

Course

How do I remember what the radial nerve supplies?

I would like to **extend** a *radiant* thank you for buying this book. (The **radial** nerve predominantly supplies the **extensors** of the arm.)

THE ULNAR NERVE

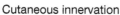

☞ Medial cord of the brachial plexus, C8 and T1.
☞ Medial to axillary artery.
☞ Travels anterior to triceps.
☞ Pierces intermuscular septum distally in the arm to enter the posterior compartment of the arm.
☞ Between medial humeral epicondyle and the olecranon, lying in the ulnar groove.
☞ Enters anterior compartment lying between two heads of flexor carpi ulnaris (FCU).
☞ Descends forearm lying on flexor digitorum profundus (FDP) and is covered by FCU belly.

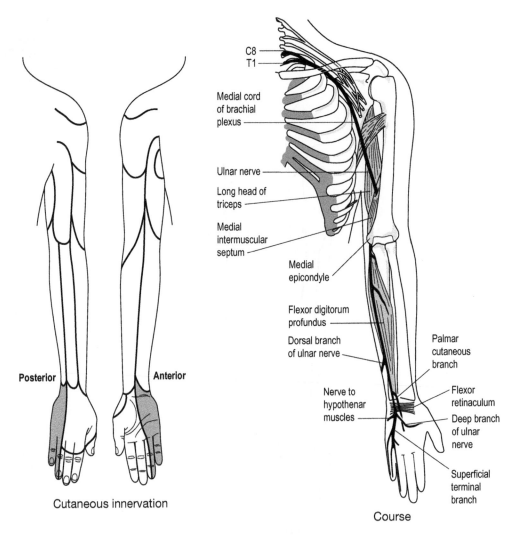

C8
T1

Medial cord
of brachial
plexus

Ulnar nerve

Long head of
triceps

Medial
intermuscular
septum

Medial
epicondyle

Flexor digitorum
profundus

Dorsal branch
of ulnar nerve

Palmar
cutaneous
branch

Nerve to
hypothenar
muscles

Flexor
retinaculum

Deep branch
of ulnar
nerve

Superficial
terminal
branch

Posterior   **Anterior**

Cutaneous innervation

Course

The ulnar nerve supplies:

☞ FCU
☞ medial half of FDP
☞ palmaris brevis
☞ hypothenar muscles
☞ medial two lumbricals
☞ adductor pollicis
☞ flexor pollicis brevis

Sensory supply is to the palmar and dorsal aspect of little finger and half of ring fingers.

Injury to ulnar nerve (claw hand) leads to hyperextension of the 4/5th MCP joints and flexion of the IP joint. The little finger drifts into abduction and the hypothenar muscles atrophy.

Question: You bang your 'funny bone' on a chair. This sends pins and needles down the medial border of your forearm, your little finger and half of your ring finger also get pins and needles.

1. Which nerve have you hit?
2. Whereabouts have you compressed the nerve on its course?

3. What is paraesthesia?
4. What is anaesthesia?
5. What is hyperaesthesia?

Answers
1. Ulnar nerve.
2. Posterior elbow between medial epicondyle and olecranon.
3. Abnormal sensation.
4. Absence of sensation.
5. Overly sensitive.

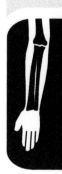

For each of the nerves in this chapter, make sure that you are able to describe the:

Motor loss

Sensory loss

Functional loss

Typical deformities

commonly resulting from paralysis of each nerve of the upper limb.

Make sure that you can demonstrate the dermatomes and myotomes of the upper limb.

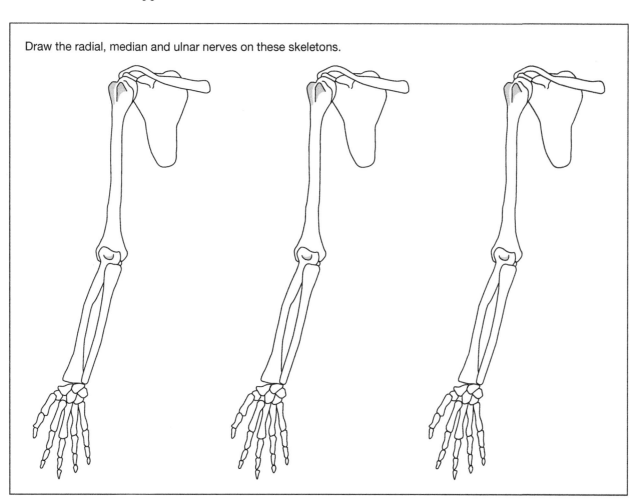

Draw the radial, median and ulnar nerves on these skeletons.

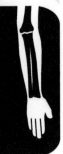

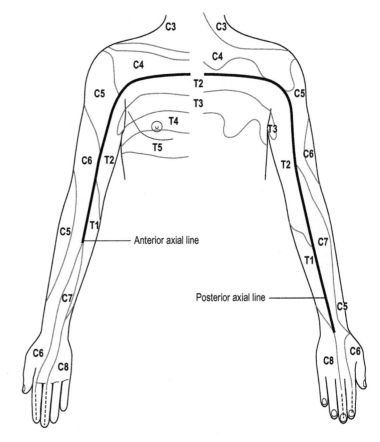

Dermatomes of the
upper limb

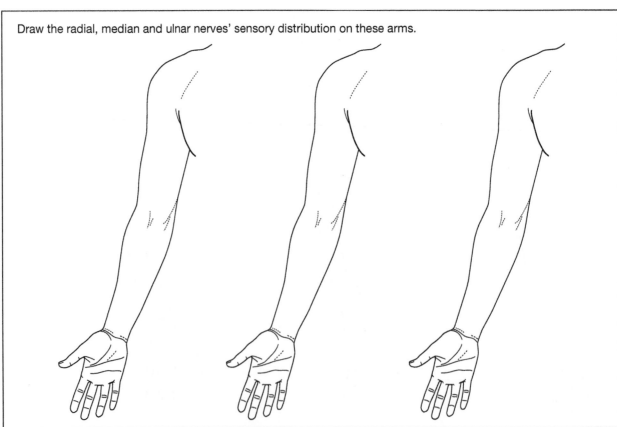

Draw the radial, median and ulnar nerves' sensory distribution on these arms.

Draw the dermatomes of the upper limb on this arm.

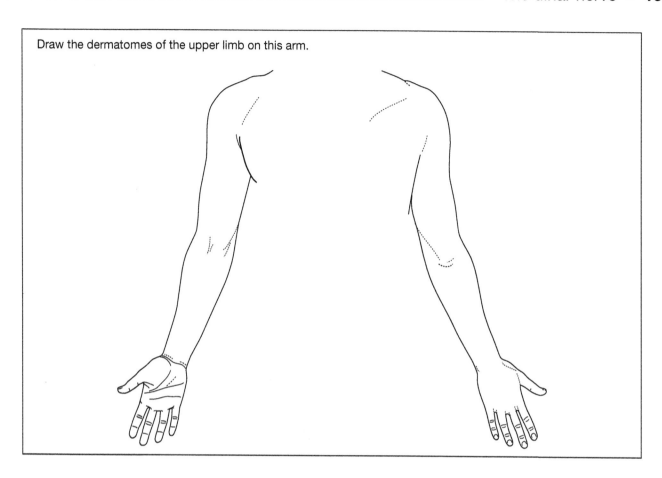

Judgement time

For the nerves of the upper limb can you describe

root level

relations

major branches

innervations

signs and symptoms resulting from lesions of the nerves listed below:

- ❏ musculocutaneous nerve
- ❏ axillary nerve
- ❏ median nerve
- ❏ ulnar nerve
- ❏ radial nerve.

Do you know the dermatomes of the upper limb?

PART

3

The spine

Learning outcomes

After reading this chapter you should be able to:

1. Describe a typical cervical, thoracic and lumbar vertebra.

2. Describe the structure and function of an intervertebral disc.

3. Describe the structure and function of the sacroiliac joint.

4. Describe the structure and function of the human spinal column.

5. Describe the articulations of the human spine.

6. Describe the following spinal ligaments:
   - Alar
   - Transverse
   - Ligamentum nuchae
   - Ligamentum flavum
   - Anterior longitudinal ligament
   - Posterior longitudinal ligament
   - Interspinous ligament
   - Supraspinous ligament.

7. Know which major muscles act on the spine.

Medicine has worked hard to get to grips with the human spine. As long ago as the 17th century BC, the ancient Egyptians were looking at the spine. One papyrus described the difference between cervical sprain, fracture and fracture-dislocation (Sanan & Rengachary 1996).

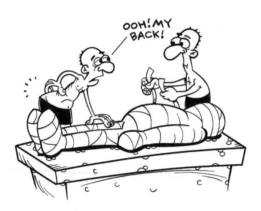

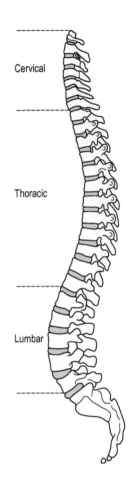

Cervical

Thoracic

Lumbar

THE BONES

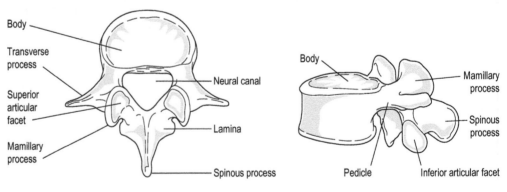

Body

Transverse process

Superior articular facet

Mamillary process

Neural canal

Lamina

Spinous process

Body

Mamillary process

Spinous process

Pedicle

Inferior articular facet

A lumbar vertebra

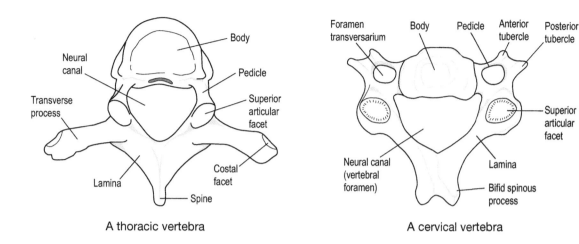

A thoracic vertebra   A cervical vertebra

It would be a worthwhile exercise to make a summary of the similarities and differences between cervical, thoracic and lumbar vertebrae, including how each is specialised and why.

The atlas and the axis

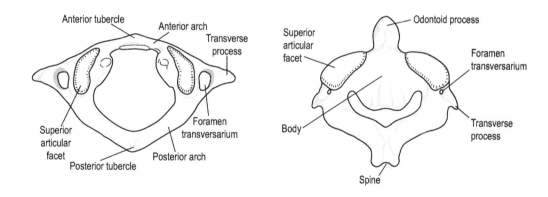

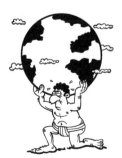

These are the names given to the first and second cervical vertebrae.

Atlas = C1. Axis = C2.

Atlas was the Greek God who it was believed supported the universe on his shoulders. In anatomical terms, the atlas supports the head. These bones are not shaped like their other fellow vertebrae.

Look at this picture:

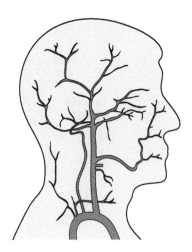

☞ Can you now work out what travels through the holes in either side of the cervical vertebrae? – that's right, it is a pair of arteries that go up towards the brain.

☞ Blockage or narrowing of the vertebral artery can lead to vertebrobasilar insufficiency (VBI); in other words lightheadedness or fainting upon certain neck movements. This is an important concept in examination and assessment of the spine.

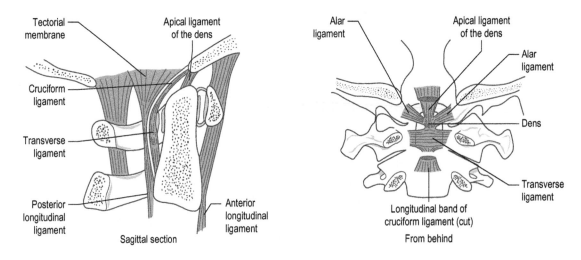

Atlanto–axial articulation

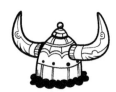

The alar ligaments basically join the odontoid to the skull. Think of them as the horns on a Viking's helmet!

Stop press … I was informed after the first edition of this book that Viking helmets didn't in fact have horns – but I'm sorry I'm not changing it now!

THE STRUCTURE OF THE SPINE

The important thing about the human spine is that it is very flexible and also very stable. It achieves this by having many individual joints, each of which only moves a small amount, but add them all together and they form a mobile structure.

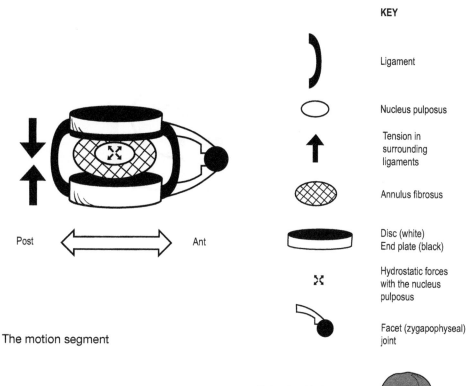

The motion segment

KEY

Ligament

Nucleus pulposus

Tension in surrounding ligaments

Annulus fibrosus

Disc (white)
End plate (black)

Hydrostatic forces with the nucleus pulposus

Facet (zygapophyseal) joint

The spine allows support and movement of the skull, flexion of the neck and back, anchor sites for the ribs, and support and protection for the spinal cord. It consists of seven cervical vertebrae, 12 thoracic vertebrae, and five lumbar vertebrae. It ends inferiorly at the sacrum, a bone made of five fused vertebrae which anchors the spine to the pelvic girdle, and the coccyx. Between each vertebra is an intervertebral disc made of cartilage, which acts as a shock absorber, to cushion the vertebral column from trauma. The disc also maintains the stability of the spinal column and yet permits small movements between two adjacent vertebrae. Intervertebral discs are like lecturers – they have a hard exterior but a soft squishy centre!

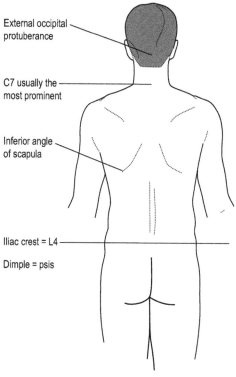

External occipital protuberance

C7 usually the most prominent

Inferior angle of scapula

Iliac crest = L4

Dimple = psis

Surface anatomy of the spine

Like a doughnut between two bricks, the disc has a vertebra above and below it. Together, these make up the so-called 'motion segment'.

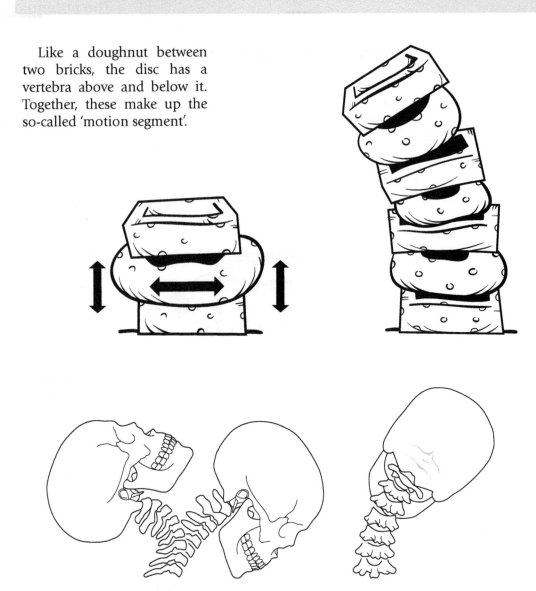

The soft-centred doughnut

The disc consists of an outer ring known as the annulus fibrosus and a gel-like portion called the nucleus pulposus. (The analogy to a jam doughnut works well.) Intervertebral discs contain fibrocytes and chondrocytes in elaborate avascular matrices of collagen and proteoglycans (Guiot & Fessler 2000). The resulting column is remarkably stable and mobile in equal proportions. The disc is pre-stressed by tension in the surrounding ligaments and the nucleus acts hydrostatically during loading. The intervertebral discs tend to become thicker as you descend the spinal column, and they tend to be wedge-shaped. The combined effect of these multiple wedges is to give the spine its three curvatures when viewed laterally. The curvatures in the cervical, lumbar and thoracic spine add to the strength of the spine and its ability to withstand compression; this also means that the line of gravity weaves anterior and posterior to the discs. The normal disc is remarkably strong and resilient to compressive loading and twisting movements, to the extent that falls from a height will often cause fracture of the vertebral body itself rather than damage to the disc.

Table 9.1

Key	Comments
E = end plates	– Permit osmosis of substances in and out of the disc – Protect the vertebra from pressure – Anchor the disc
N = nucleus pulposus	– Type 11 collagen only – Hydrophilic (likes to absorb water) – Kept in check by the annulus
A = annulus fibrosus	– Type 1 collagen (typical of tendon) provides the disc with tensile strength – Type 11 collagen (typical of cartilage) provides the disc with compressive strength

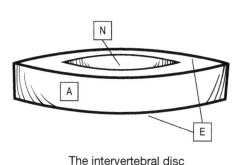

The intervertebral disc

The inelastic envelope provided by the annulus fibrosus (the fibres of which have a criss-cross arrangement of collagen bundles) restrains the nucleus. It has been known for some time that the outer portion of the annulus possesses nerve endings mainly in the outer (lateral) half of the annulus fibrosus, and hence may produce pain (Yoshizawa *et al.* 1980). This may explain the presence of back symptoms which occur even when discs appear intact and normal (Bogduk 1991).

Above and below each disc is the end plate. This has several functions: it permits osmosis from the vertebral body both in and out of the disc, it restrains the disc and it may protect the vertebrae from pressure.

It can be difficult to visualise how things are put together in the spine, so try this exercise. Make your own 'tasty' spinal column. This spinal column can only help you to lose weight as part of a calorie-controlled diet.

In this analogy, the disc sits on top and underneath each marshmallow, the spinal cord runs through the polo mint. Compare your finished model to the diagrams in the book, and make sure you understand and can name the parts of the vertebra, then eat your model.

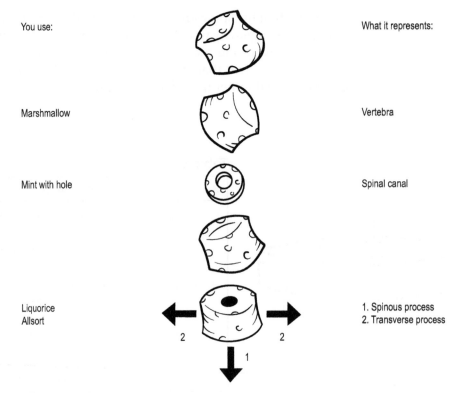

You use:		What it represents:
Marshmallow		Vertebra
Mint with hole		Spinal canal
Liquorice Allsort		1. Spinous process 2. Transverse process

The facet joints

The orientation of the facet joints controls the direction and amount of movement possible in the spine. For example, in the thoracic spine, they are aligned in such a way as to permit free rotation.

This is not the case in the lumbar spine where they are arranged so as to limit rotation. See the diagrams below.

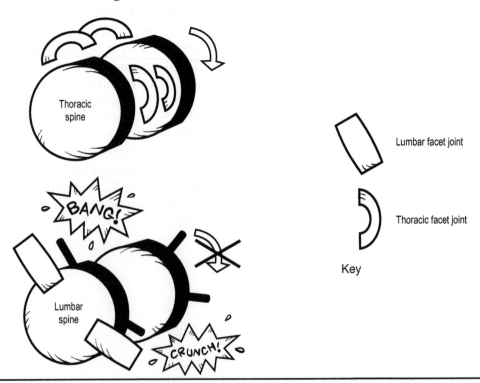

The facet joints (zygapophyseal joints)

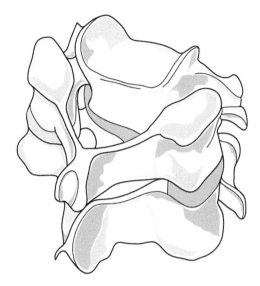

☞ How are facet joints arranged in the cervical spine?
☞ What are they?
☞ Where are they?
☞ What is their function?

The uncovertebral joints

☞ What are they?
☞ Where are they?

These are also called the joints of Luschka, or the neurocentral joints; they consist of articulations in the five lower cervical vertebral bodies, formed by the space between one vertebral body and the uncinate processes that project from the vertebral body immediately below it.

The ligaments of the spine

☞ Anterior longitudinal ligament (1 overleaf).
☞ Posterior longitudinal ligament (3 overleaf).
☞ Intertransverse ligament (2 overleaf).
☞ Interspinous ligament (4 overleaf).
☞ Supraspinous ligament (5 overleaf).
☞ Ligamentum nuchae (self-directed).
☞ Ligamentum flavum (self-directed).

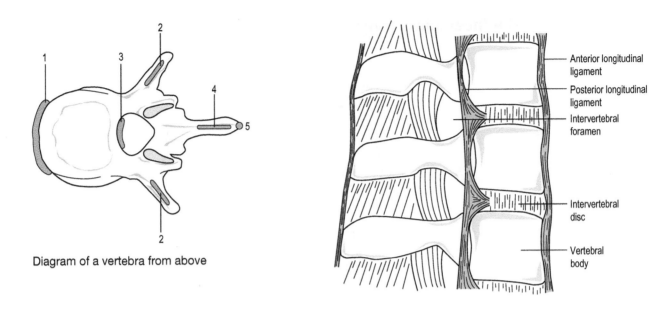

Diagram of a vertebra from above

For each of the ligaments on this diagram complete the table.

Table 9.2

Ligament	Attachments	Function
Supraspinous		
Ligamentum flavum		
Anterior longitudinal		
Posterior longitudinal		
Interspinous		

THE MUSCLES OF THE SPINE

The abdominal muscles

☞ Rectus abdominis.
☞ Internal oblique.
☞ External oblique.
☞ Transversus abdominis.

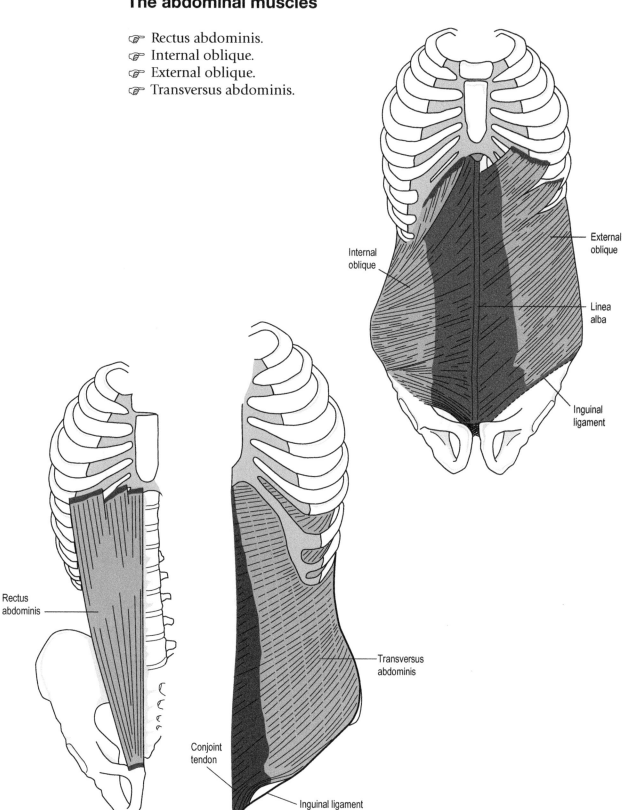
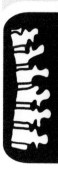

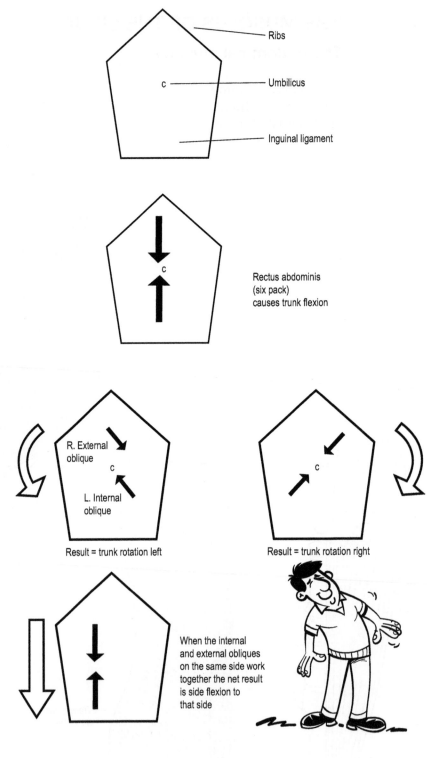

Ribs

Umbilicus

Inguinal ligament

Rectus abdominis
(six pack)
causes trunk flexion

R. External
oblique

L. Internal
oblique

Result = trunk rotation left

Result = trunk rotation right

When the internal
and external obliques
on the same side work
together the net result
is side flexion to
that side

Muscles flexing the trunk

Complete this table:

Table 9.3

Name	Origin	Insertion	Action	Function
Rectus abdominis				
External oblique				
Internal oblique				
Psoas major/minor				

Muscles extending the trunk

Complete this table:

Table 9.4

Name	Origin	Insertion	Action	Function
Quadratus lumborum				
Multifidus				
Semispinalis				
Erector spinae				

Erector spinae

This is a complex of muscles which has origins on the sacrum and lumbar spine. It passes upwards and splits into three bundles:

☞ Iliocostalis
☞ Spinalis
☞ Longissimus.

What does it do?

☞ It extends the trunk
☞ It resists flexion
☞ It helps maintain the lordosis.

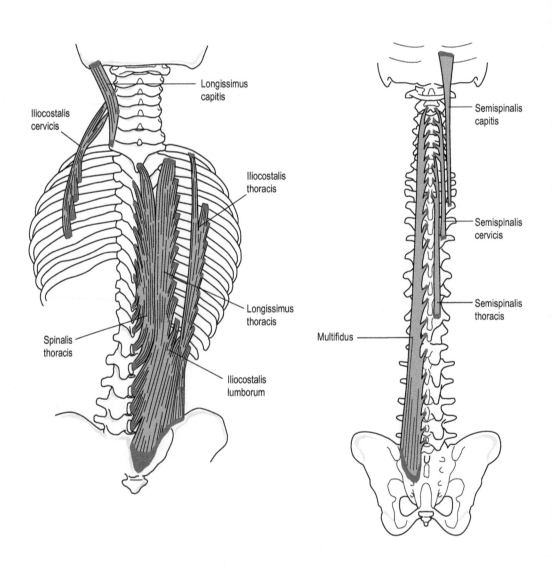

THE INTERVERTEBRAL DISC AND ITS PATHOLOGY

A normal intervertebral disc is crucial if normal motion of the human spine is to occur (Thompson *et al.* 2000).

Think of the disc in this way.

The discs of a baby are like squash balls.

The discs of an adult are like jam doughnuts, soft centred with a hard outside.

The disc of an 80-year-old is like a popadum, dry and brittle.

STRUCTURE

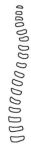

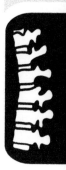

Intervertebral disc pathology

A normal disc has a hard outer rim called an annulus and a soft pulpy or gel-like centre called a nucleus.

The disc is normally hydrophilic (water-loving). You are taller when you wake up in the morning because the disc absorbs water overnight as you lie down.

With age it becomes less hydrophilic and loses height as it desiccates (dries out).

Discs get thicker as one descends the column (they have to carry more weight) and they help to contribute towards the spinal curves.

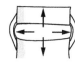

In a normal disc, stresses and strains are evenly distributed throughout the disc. The disc is so strong that a fall from a height will often fracture the vertebra itself rather than burst the disc. Healthy discs are water-loving (hydrophilic) and swell, pushing adjacent vertebrae apart, tightening surrounding ligaments.

The disc lies in close proximity to the spinal cord, nerve roots and intervertebral foramina.

The function of the discs is to give each segment stability with a small degree of mobility. When all the spinal column movements are added together, the spine is very mobile but retains its stability.

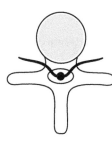

Repeated flexed postures or trauma places massive stress on the posterior of the disc, this may cause the nucleus to herniate or bulge, like the jam leaking out of a jam doughnut. Sometimes a piece of disc breaks off and floats around. This is sequestration.

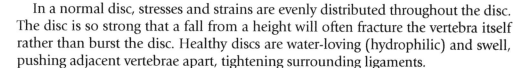

Schmorl's nodes

Occasionally, the disc herniates through the end plate itself. This is called a Schmorl's node.

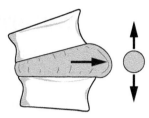

Schmorl's node

Prolapsed intervertebral disc (PID)

Because of the anatomy of surrounding ligaments, most protrusions are posterolateral (back and to one side). The significance of this is that the adjacent nerve root may become inflamed or 'trapped'. This will result in referred pain in the distribution of the corresponding nerve supply. A large or central bulge may cause spinal cord compression, and so-called long tract signs such as loss of bowel and bladder control and spasticity.

Lumbar spondylosis (disc degeneration or wear and tear)

Along with prolapse, this is probably the most common spinal condition. The disc loses height with age. It is less good at taking stresses and strains and spinal movement diminishes. Because of this loss of joint space, more strain is put on the facet joints, causing them to degenerate.

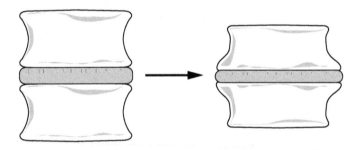

Professor asks

If the disc itself has virtually no nerve supply, why should a prolapsed intervertebral disc give a patient so much pain?

Clues:
Think about the surrounding structures.
Think about the by-products of the inflammatory process.

Answer
It is not only the mechanical pressure from the disc that causes pain, the inflammatory reaction in the area also causes pain and irritation of the surrounding nerve roots.

Why are anterior protrusions relatively asymptomatic?
Clue: what structures are anterior in the spinal column?

Why are most protrusions in a posterolateral direction, as the one shown above?
Clue: which ligament lies posterior to the disc and would therefore tend to resist posterior disc displacement?

THE SACROILIAC JOINT

☞ Where is it? It is an L-shaped joint between the ilium and the ala of the sacrum roughly marked out as a line from the posterior superior iliac spine (PSIS) running 25° superolaterally to inferomedially 2.5 cm either way from the PSIS.

☞ How is it classified? The weird thing is that it is partly synovial and partly fibrous.

☞ The main ligaments are anterior and posterior.

☞ How much movement occurs at this joint? Depends who you ask! Wang & Dumas (1998) did studies on cadavers and claim that 'Lateral rotation and nutation rotation of the sacrum were found to be the predominant motion, though the values were limited to less than 1.2°. Both the anterior and posterior sacroiliac ligaments were found to play an important role in resisting rotations at the joints.'

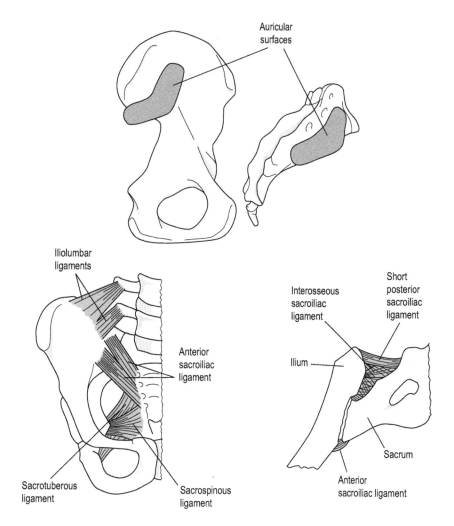

The sacroiliac joint

DEGENERATIVE SPINAL DISORDERS AT A GLANCE

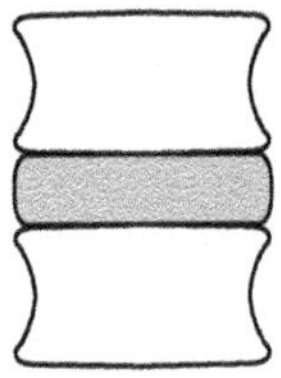

Normal spine

Your notes

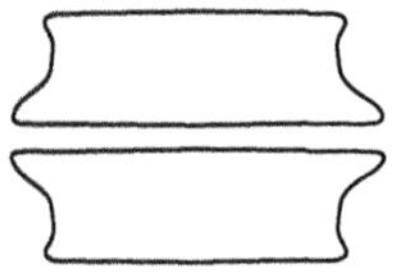

_____

_____

_____

_____

_____

_____

_____

Spondylosis

Your notes

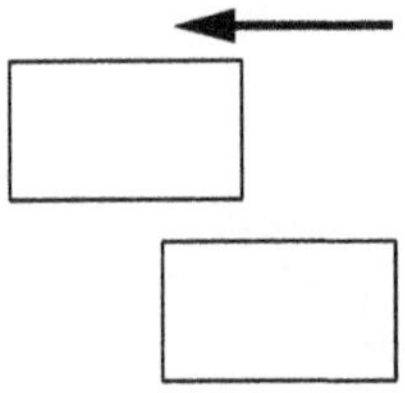

_____

_____

_____

_____

_____

_____

_____

_____

Spondylolisthesis

Your notes

_____

_____

_____

_____

_____

_____

_____

Judgement time

Can you:

1. Describe a typical cervical, thoracic and lumbar vertebra?
2. Describe the structure and function of an intervertebral disc?
3. Describe the structure and function of the sacroiliac joint?
4. Describe the structure and function of the human spinal column?
5. Describe the articulations of the human spine?
6. Describe these ligaments?
   - ❑ Alar
   - ❑ Transverse
   - ❑ Ligamentum nuchae
   - ❑ Ligamentum flavum
   - ❑ Anterior longitudinal ligament
   - ❑ Posterior longitudinal ligament
   - ❑ Interspinous ligament
   - ❑ Supraspinous ligament.
7. Do you have knowledge of the major muscles acting on the spine?

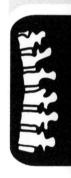

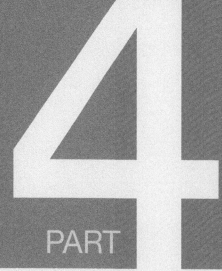

PART

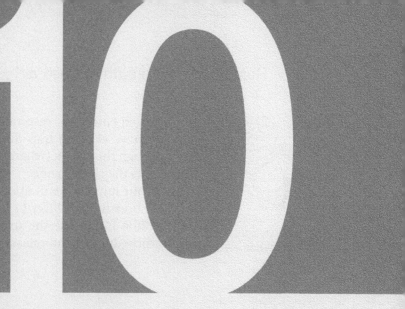

CHAPTER

Respiration – a breath of fresh air!

Learning outcomes

By the end of this chapter, you will have an understanding of

1. The gross structure of the lungs, their major lobes and the bronchial tree.

2. The structure of the alveoli.

3. The functions of the diaphragm.

4. How the ribs move during respiration.

5. The location and function of the pleura.

6. What caused the mummy's curse (just checking you're paying attention!).

Single-celled organisms don't need a respiratory system; they can rely on their one and only cell membrane to allow oxygen and other things in and out – the simple life. Several million years ago, however, our ancestors decided that they needed more cells and as a result we had to think up a system of keeping them fed. We now need a complex system of vessels, tubes and other organs to do this job. The respiratory system's job is to supply oxygen to all parts of the body and get rid of what we don't want. The respiratory system does this through breathing. When we breathe, we inhale oxygen and exhale carbon dioxide. This exchange of gases is how the respiratory system gets oxygen into the blood.

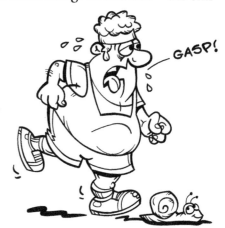

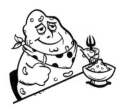

Survival for the amoebas – a simple affair.

Oxygen enters our respiratory system through our mouth and nose. The hairs in the nose (YUCK) trap dust and warm the air a little. The oxygen then passes through the larynx (where speech sounds are made) and the trachea – a tube that enters the chest cavity.

Your lungs contain about 2400 km (1500 miles) of airways and every minute you breathe in 6 litres (13 pints) of air. Plants are our partners in breathing. We breathe in air, use the oxygen in it, and release carbon dioxide. Plants take in carbon dioxide and release oxygen.

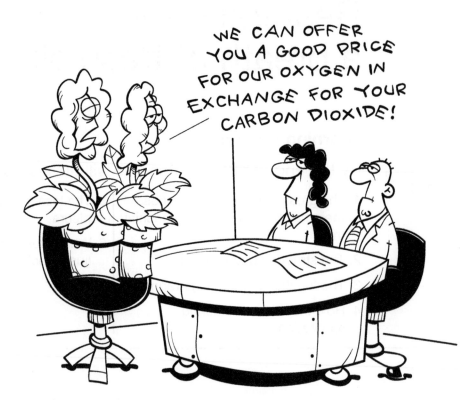

A fair deal if you ask me!

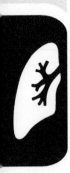

THE BRONCHIAL TREE

The respiratory system is often described as a tree – the bronchial tree to be exact, and just like trees have a single trunk which then splits into progressively smaller and smaller branches so does the respiratory system. There may be as many as 28 progressively smaller divisions of the bronchial tree beyond the point where the trachea (windpipe) splits. The proximal divisions are involved with getting the air in and out whilst the distal divisions are where the important job of gas exchange happens.

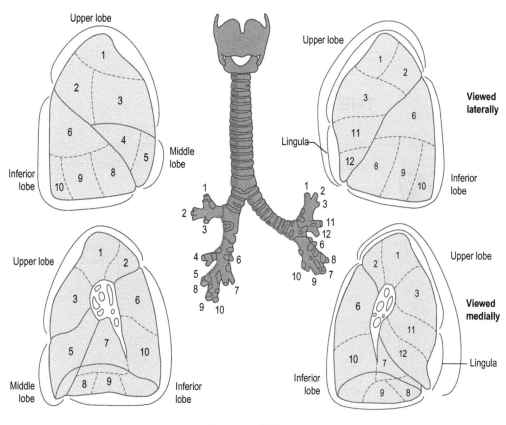

The bronchial tree

THE TRACHEA (THE WINDPIPE)

The trachea is a tube. Like the attachment on your vacuum cleaner it needs to be kept open so it is reinforced by 15–20 regularly spaced cartilages which are C shaped; behind the trachea is the oesophagus or food pipe.

On the diagram, colour in the trachea, its rings and the oesophagus so you understand where each is located.

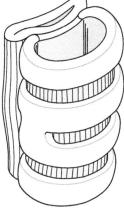

Trachea

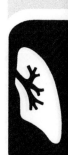

The trachea is in your neck just below your cricoid cartilage. This is the about the same level as the sixth cervical vertebra.

THE LUNGS

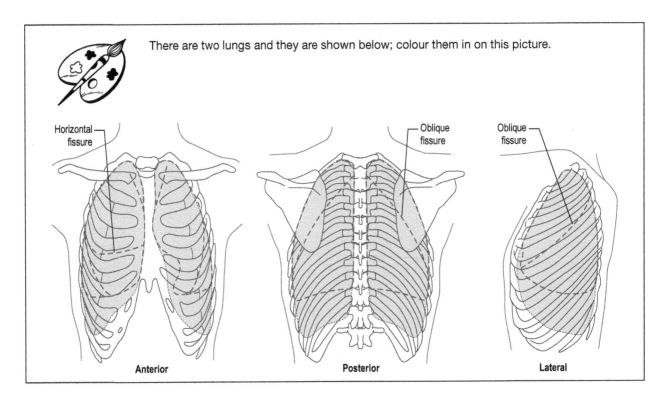

There are two lungs and they are shown below; colour them in on this picture.

Horizontal fissure

Oblique fissure

Oblique fissure

Anterior

Posterior

Lateral

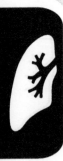

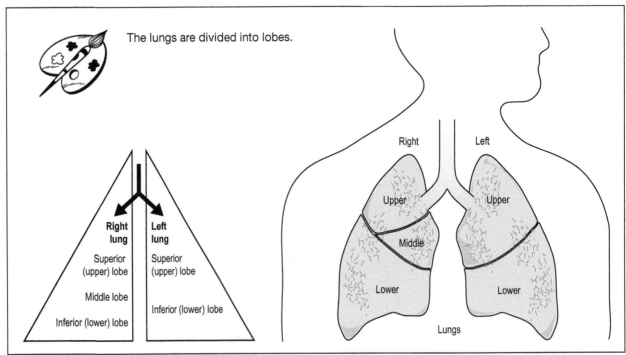

The lungs are divided into lobes.

Right lung

Superior (upper) lobe

Middle lobe

Inferior (lower) lobe

Left lung

Superior (upper) lobe

Inferior (lower) lobe

Right

Left

Upper

Upper

Middle

Lower

Lower

Lungs

The end of the line

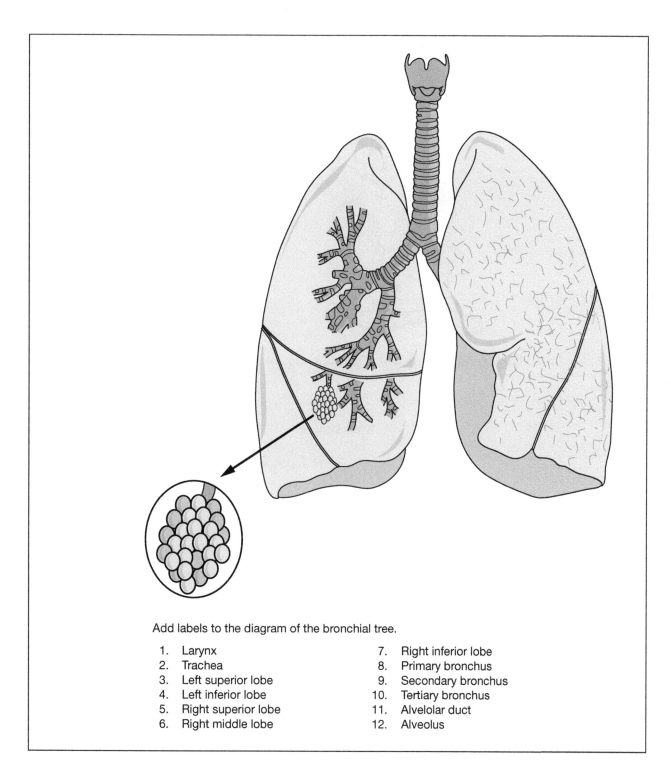

Add labels to the diagram of the bronchial tree.

1. Larynx
2. Trachea
3. Left superior lobe
4. Left inferior lobe
5. Right superior lobe
6. Right middle lobe
7. Right inferior lobe
8. Primary bronchus
9. Secondary bronchus
10. Tertiary bronchus
11. Alvelolar duct
12. Alveolus

Think of the bronchial tree as a motorway (the trachea) which splits into two main roads (the left and right main bronchi) and then into avenues, and then the last roads – the cul de sacs if you will, are the alveoli. The walls of these are very thin and moist which allows gases to easily pass through. The surfaces of the alveoli are covered with capillaries which allow the gases to come into close contact with the alveolar walls then therefore either get in or out depending on what we need. Alveoli are smaller than a grain of sand and there are about 300 million of them in the lungs. Alveoli have a very large surface area in total like the clown with his balloons below.

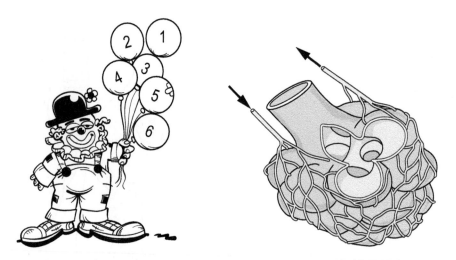

Look at this picture which shows you how gases move in and out of the alveoli.

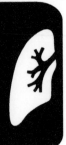

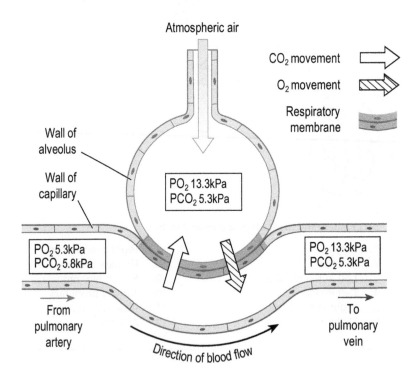

MAKING BREATHING HAPPEN

How do we get air in and out?

The diaphragm is the main inspiration muscle. It's a thin and parachute-shaped sheet and it inserts into your lower ribs. When it contracts, it pushes downward and spreads out, increasing the vertical dimension of the chest cavity and driving up pressure in the abdomen. This drives the abdominal contents down and out, which in turn increases the transverse size of the chest cavity.

When the diaphragm contracts it pulls the pleura down with it. This lowers the pleural pressure, which causes alveolar pressure to drop, which, in turn, causes air to be sucked into the lungs. During quiet expiration, the diaphragm relaxes and returns to where it started. BUT, during exercise, expiration becomes much more of an active process: the external intercostal muscles (the bits you eat when you have spare ribs in a restaurant or takeaway!) raise the lower ribs up and out, increasing the sideways and front to back dimensions of the thorax. The scalene muscles and sternocleidomastoid also get busy, raising and pushing out the upper ribs and the sternum. The abdominals contract to raise the pressure in the abdomen, which pushes the diaphragm upward and forces air out of the lungs. The rib cage is not rigid whilst all this is going on, the ribs are joined to the spine at the thorax at the back and as you breathe in they flare outwards like the handle on a bucket being lifted up – not surprisingly called bucket handle movement.

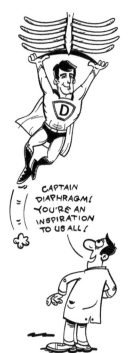

CAPTAIN DIAPHRAGM! YOU'RE AN INSPIRATION TO US ALL!

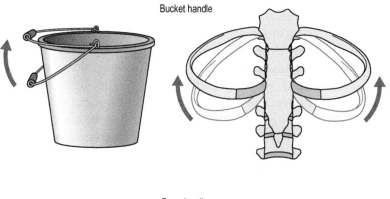

Bucket handle

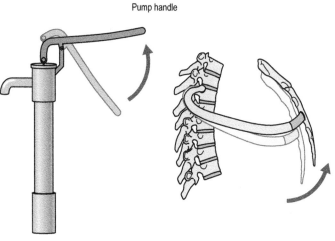

Pump handle

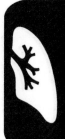

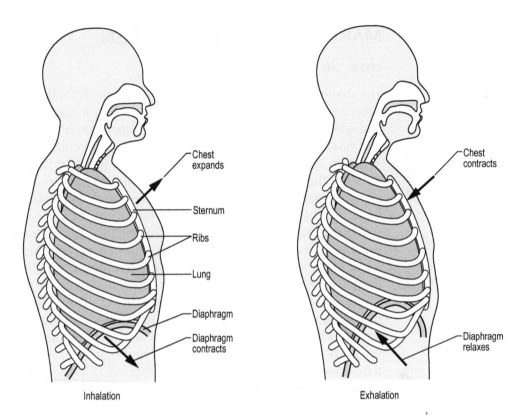

Chest
expands

Sternum

Ribs

Lung

Diaphragm

Diaphragm
contracts

Inhalation

Chest
contracts

Diaphragm
relaxes

Exhalation

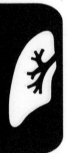

Now, remember bursae? Well just to refresh your memory these are nature's anti-friction devices and we have them wherever there is a lot of movement, so think about breathing for a while. It's something that you have more or less been continuously doing since the day that you were born, so we need to keep wear and tear down to a minimum. To help with this we have two membranes, called pleura, that line the lungs. The visceral and parietal pleura are smooth and secrete fluid, which occupies the space between them; this space is termed the pleural cavity. The fluid permits free movement of the lungs as they expand and contract during respiration. The pleura may be affected by a range of conditions, e.g. infection (pleurisy) and malignancy (mesothelioma), trapped air (pneumothorax), pus (empyema) and blood (haemothorax).

Here they are:

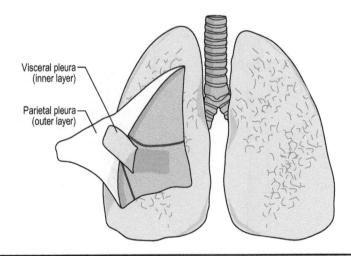

Visceral pleura
(inner layer)

Parietal pleura
(outer layer)

On the picture below, colour in the pleural space.

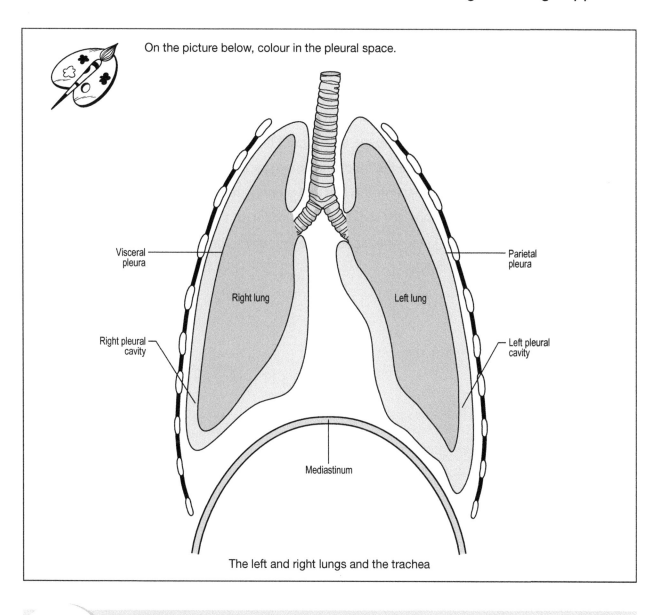

The left and right lungs and the trachea

Attacking your lungs ... from beyond the grave
Bet you thought the curse of King Tut was a myth — well think
again. Recent studies have shown that some ancient tombs do
indeed carry dormant moulds and spores including the species
Aspergillus niger and Aspergillus flavus. These bugs lie dormant
alongside the mummy and in the tomb until an unsuspecting
archaeologist comes along and breaks into the tomb. The spores then
reawaken and are inhaled, attacking the tissues in the lungs. They
can cause allergic reactions ranging from pulmonary congestion
to bleeding in the lungs. Scientists have also detected ammonia,
and hydrogen sulphide, inside sealed mummy coffins. In strong
concentrations these cause burning in the eyes, nose and throat,
pneumonia-like symptoms, and in extreme cases ... death.

Scared ... ?

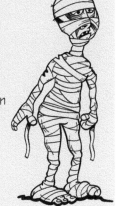
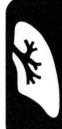

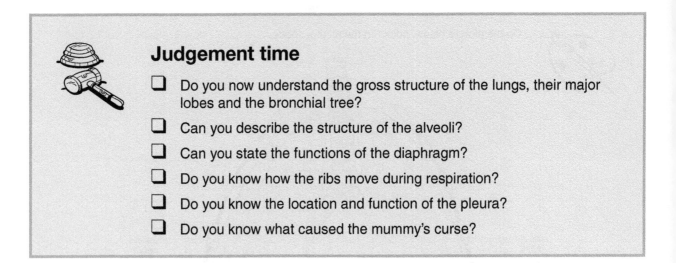

Judgement time

❏ Do you now understand the gross structure of the lungs, their major lobes and the bronchial tree?

❏ Can you describe the structure of the alveoli?

❏ Can you state the functions of the diaphragm?

❏ Do you know how the ribs move during respiration?

❏ Do you know the location and function of the pleura?

❏ Do you know what caused the mummy's curse?

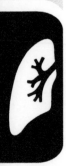

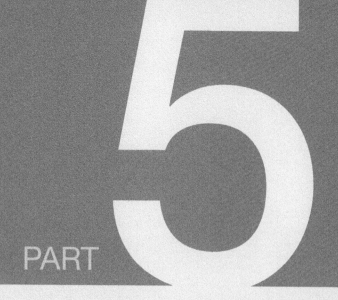

PART

The brain and nervous system

'It is in the brain that everything takes place .... It is in the brain that the poppy is red, that the apple is odorous, that the skylark sings'

Oscar Wilde

Learning outcomes

After reading this chapter you should be able to:

1. Describe the structure of the brain and spinal cord.

2. Know how the nervous system, meninges and ventricles are organised.

3. Know what neuroplasticity is.

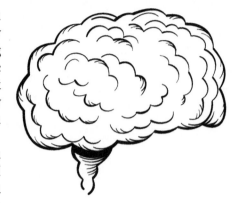

According to the ancient Egyptians, the brain had no significance in the human body; they believed that your heart did all the thinking so they left this in place after you died. The brain was thought to be so unimportant that it was removed in pieces and thrown away after death, since it wouldn't be needed in the afterlife – big mistake.

I remember when I was a student back in the 1980s (a fantastic decade by the way) I went to the medical school and held a human brain in my hands. Having done this, I can understand why the Egyptians thought the brain was nothing special. The human brain is greyish and is about the size of a cauliflower (mine is considerably larger – more like a melon, according to my wife).

We now know that the ancients were wrong and that the brain is where we 'exist'. It has its own system of cables and junction boxes to allow our bodies to do what they need to do.

WHAT DO OUR BRAIN AND NERVOUS SYSTEM DO?

Senses

The brain detects changes in our environment: e.g. when it is cold, the brain tells us to shiver – the heat generated by our muscles keeps our bodies at normal temperature

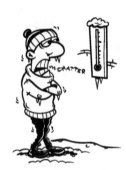

Integrates

The brain analyses sensory input, stores information and decides on the best response, e.g. the fight or flight response.

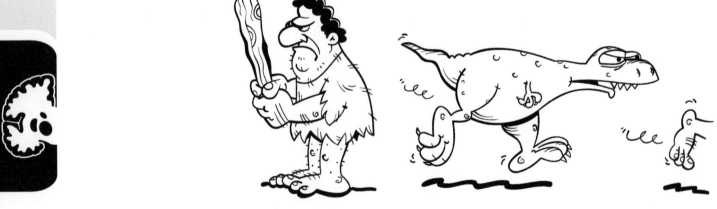

Fight   or flight

Movement

The brain is responsible for our movement – life would be dull indeed if we couldn't move.

Your nervous system is organised as follows:

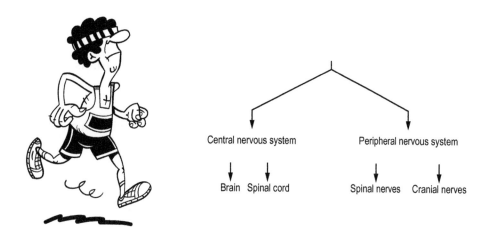

This is how your brain looks from the side. On the picture colour in the cerebrum, brainstem and cerebellum.

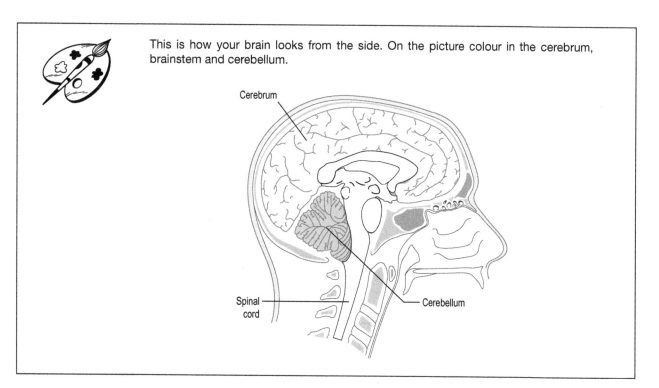

Let's think about the brain first of all. There are one hundred billion neurons in the brain. The outer surface is called the cerebral cortex; it has a grey colour because it consists of cell bodies; like a cauliflower it is crinkly on the outside, and quite delicate. So let's go through some general points and see whether we can work out what goes where and why. Beneath the cortex is the white matter (nerve cell fibres); the brain is usually divided into brainstem, midbrain and forebrain. The cauliflower itself is called the cerebrum and is in two halves, the

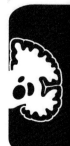

cerebral hemispheres, each of which is divided into lobes as in the picture below. There are several membranes, which act, like air bags on a car, to protect the brain; these are called the meninges and are as follows:

the **dura mater**, the **arachnoid mater**, and the **pia mater**.

Pia mater

The pia mater is a very delicate membrane. It is attached to: (nearest) the *brain* or the *spinal cord*. As such, it follows all the minor contours of the brain and it firmly adheres to the surface of the brain and spinal cord. Its *capillaries* nourish the brain.

Arachnoid mater

This has a spider-web-like appearance. It provides a cushioning effect for the *central nervous system*. The arachnoid mater exists as a thin, transparent membrane.

Dura mater

The dura mater is thick, and is closest to the *skull*. It contains larger blood vessels that split into the capillaries in the pia mater. You may encounter people who have had a bleed under this membrane – this is called a sub-dural haematoma and can be life threatening as there is nowhere for the swelling to go except inward, towards the soft, delicate brain.

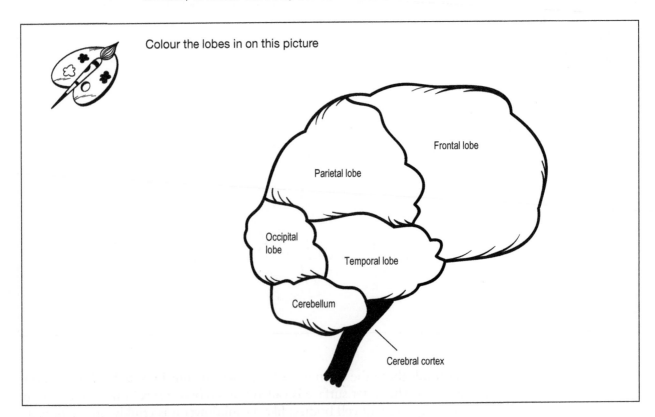

Colour the lobes in on this picture

Frontal lobe

Parietal lobe

Occipital lobe

Temporal lobe

Cerebellum

Cerebral cortex

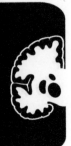

The ventricles

These are a system of four cavities within the brain that are continuous with the central canal in the spinal cord. In the same way that a car engine needs oil to lubricate, feed and protect it, the brain is bathed in fluid – cerebrospinal fluid which is produced in the ventricles.

There are two lateral ventricles, the third ventricle and the fourth ventricle.

Lateral ventricles: These sit within the cerebral hemispheres. Each consists of a triangular central body and four horns.

The third ventricle is a median cavity in the brain that is bounded by the thalamus and hypothalamus on either side.

The fourth ventricle is the most inferior of the four ventricles of the brain. It extends from the midbrain to the upper end of the spinal cord.

The ventricles are filled with cerebrospinal fluid (CSF), which is formed by the choroid plexuses in the walls and roofs of the ventricles. This fluid can be drained and examined in medicine to diagnose things like meningitis (inflammation of the meninges) or encephalitis (inflammation of the brain).

DOES HAVING A BIG BRAIN MAKE YOU CLEVER?

This is an interesting question: there is some evidence of a link between brain volume and IQ but it is not that simple. When the scientific genius Albert Einstein died in 1955 his brain was examined and it was found to be to all intents

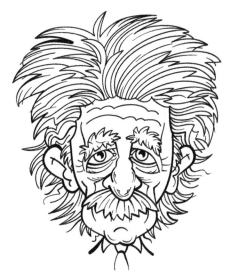

and purposes the same as any other; in fact there was one area of his brain that was missing (the parietal operculum). It may be that because of this, adjacent parts of his brain developed more (the inferior parietal lobes).

These regions are known to have something to do with visual imagery and mathematical thinking resulting in his great ability to think about abstract concepts that we all find so difficult.

Here is what Einstein had to say about his thought processes:

'I never came upon any of my discoveries through the process of rational thinking.'

Before you ask, I'm not even going to get into the argument about whether the brain of man is bigger or smaller than the brain of a woman!

DEVELOPING WHAT YOU'VE GOT – PLASTICITY

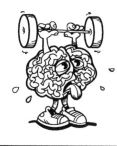

The brain is often compared to a computer – this is a fair comparison I suppose, but it does not really reflect just how fantastic the human brain is. Look at it this way – whenever my computer has gone wrong I've either had to buy a new one, install some really expensive software or throw the whole thing through the window and start again (believe me, in the time I've been writing books and doing my PhD I've got through three computers) but I'm still on brain number one.

In some respects, the brain is a little more like a muscle – use it and it responds by growing. If a human brain does something often enough, the neural pathways

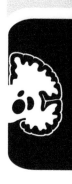

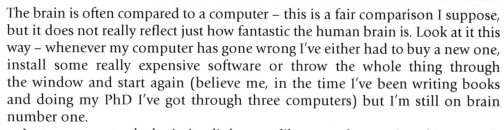

get stronger, and even more amazingly, if part of the brain is damaged it can actually re-route power to other parts which can take over; this is a little like asking your computer to fix itself by creating new programs – oh, how I wish!

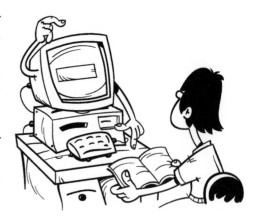

Neuroplasticity is the word that refers to these changes that occur as a result of the effect of *experience*, repetition and as a response to trauma. The main point is that our brains are not *hard-wired*.

The brainstem

The brainstem is the most primitive part of our brain and a lot of what goes on here is concerned with our survival; for example, blood pressure, breathing, digestion, heart rate and eating– the things that we need to do but the things that we don't need to think about. It is a little like a computer freeing up space on a second hard disk for important functions!

Most of the cranial nerves also come from the brainstem. The brainstem is also a type of junction box for all fibre tracts passing up and down from peripheral nerves and spinal cord to the higher centres of your brain.

More on the cranial nerves

The cranial nerves are 12 pairs of nerves that emanate from the brain. In order to reach their targets they must ultimately exit/enter the cranium through openings in the skull. They are as follows.

Write a few lines on the function of each in the space below each one

   I Olfactory nerve

   II Optic nerve

   III Oculomotor nerve

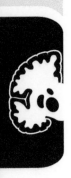

   IV Trochlear nerve

V   Trigeminal nerve

VI   Abducens nerve

VII   Facial nerve

VIII   Vestibulocochlear nerve

IX   Glossopharyngeal nerve

X   Vagus nerve

XI   Accessory nerve

XII   Hypoglossal nerve

Medulla oblongata – The medulla oblongata is as a junction box for the crossing of motor tracts between the spinal cord and the brain. It contains the respiratory, vasomotor and cardiac centres, as well as many mechanisms for controlling reflex activities such as coughing, swallowing and vomiting.

Midbrain – The midbrain serves as the nerve pathway of the cerebral hemispheres and contains auditory and visual reflex centres.

Pons – A bridge-like structure linking different parts of the brain, acting as a relay station from the medulla to the higher cortical structures of the brain. It contains the respiratory centre.

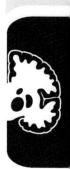

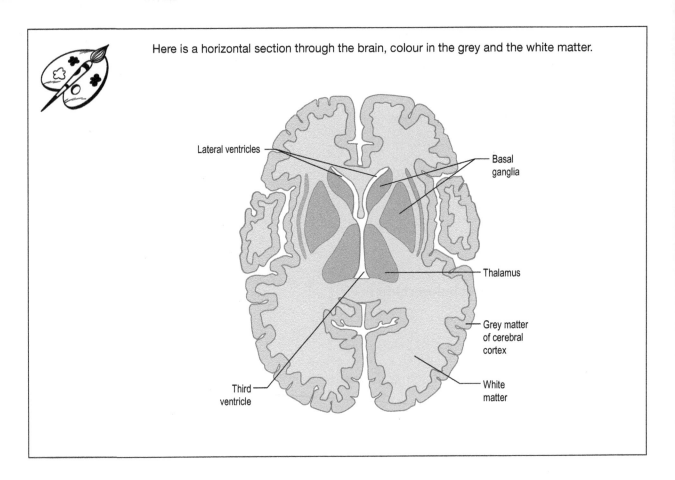

Here is a horizontal section through the brain, colour in the grey and the white matter.

Lateral ventricles

Basal ganglia

Thalamus

Grey matter of cerebral cortex

White matter

Third ventricle

The spinal cord is the motorway between your brain and the rest of your body.

☞ The spinal cord sits inside the spinal column.
☞ The spinal cord is joined with the brainstem at the top.
☞ It begins at the base of the skull, extends down to about the first or second lumbar vertebra, then from this point downwards it is a collection of bundles called the cauda equina (this means horse's tail). That is why it is safe for a doctor to do a lumbar puncture without risk of hitting the spinal cord.
☞ Sensory input in on the **dorsal side**.
☞ Muscle control output in on the **ventral side**.

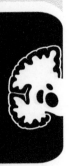

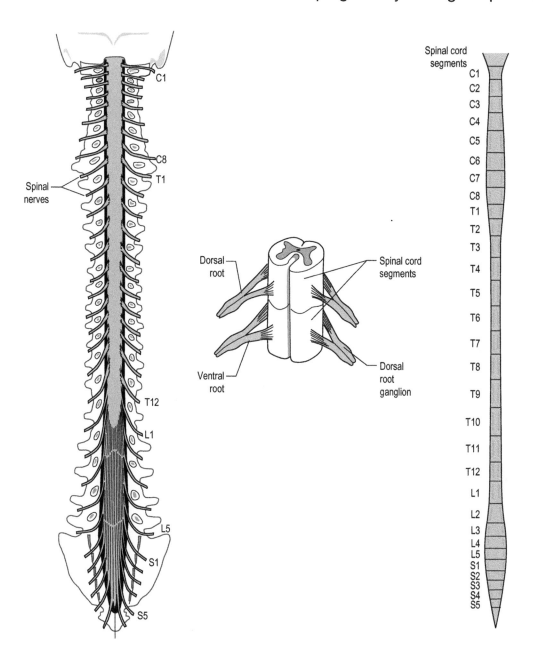

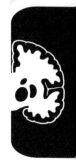

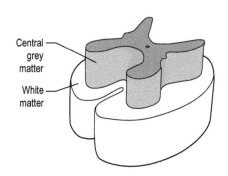

Central grey matter

White matter

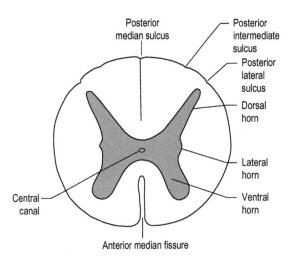

Posterior median sulcus

Posterior intermediate sulcus

Posterior lateral sulcus

Dorsal horn

Lateral horn

Ventral horn

Central canal

Anterior median fissure

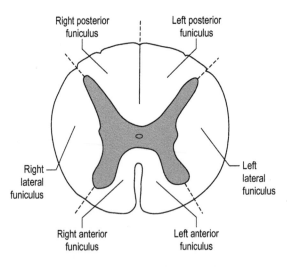

Right posterior funiculus

Left posterior funiculus

Right lateral funiculus

Left lateral funiculus

Right anterior funiculus

Left anterior funiculus

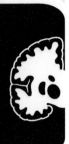

Judgement time

- ❏ Can you now describe the structure of the brain and spinal cord?
- ❏ Do you know how the nervous system, meninges and ventricles are organised?
- ❏ Do you know what neuroplasticity is?

Photographic atlas

Figure A.1

Landmarks on the lateral aspect of the leg

popliteal fossa   1
biceps femoris   2
vastus lateralis   3
patella   4
tibial tuberosity   5
lateral malleolus   6
tendons of peroneus longus and brevis   7
tendons of extensor digitorum longus   8
Achilles tendon   9
muscle belly of gastrocnemius   10
soleus   11

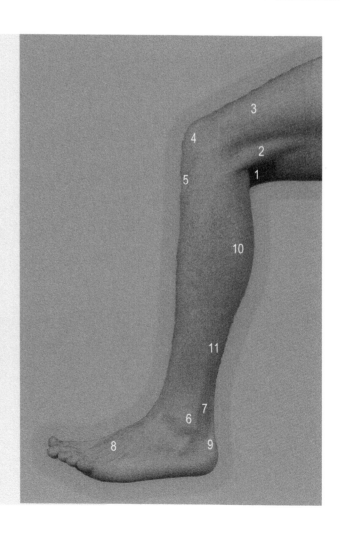

Figure A.2

Landmarks in the lower limb

anterior superior iliac spine	1
pubic tubercle	2
rectus femoris	3
vastus lateralis	4
vastus medialis	5
rectus femoris	6
patella	7
ligamentum patellae (patellar tendon)	8
tibial tuberosity	9
anterior border of tibia	10

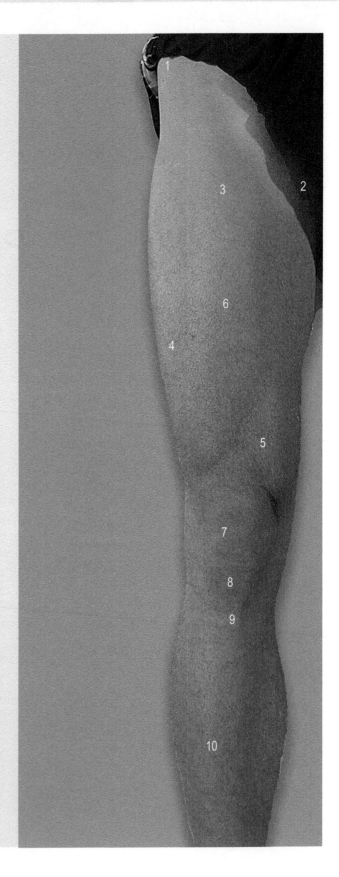

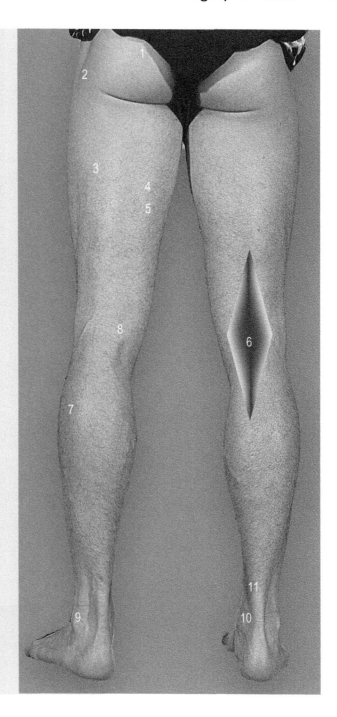

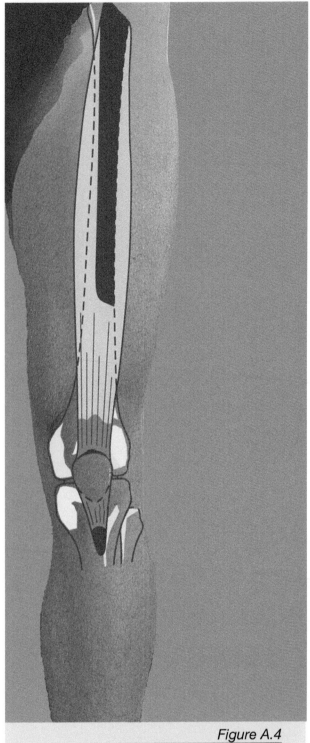

Figure A.4

Vastus intermedius

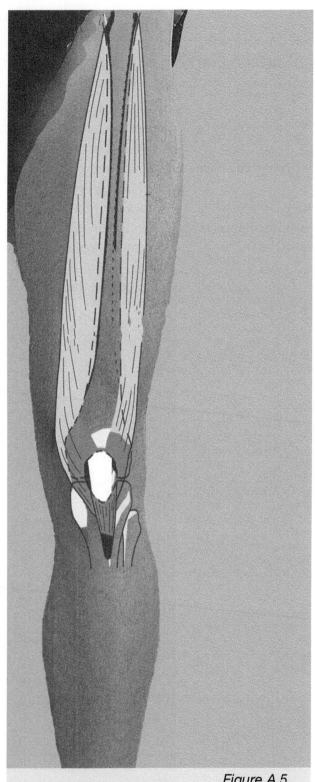

Figure A.5

Vastus medialis and vastus lateralis

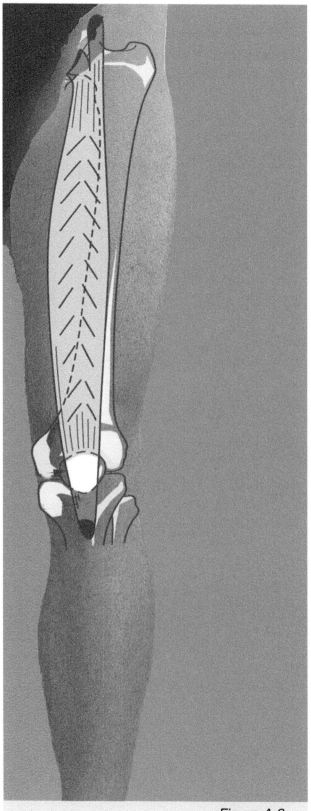

Figure A.6

Rectus femoris

Figure A.7

Q angle

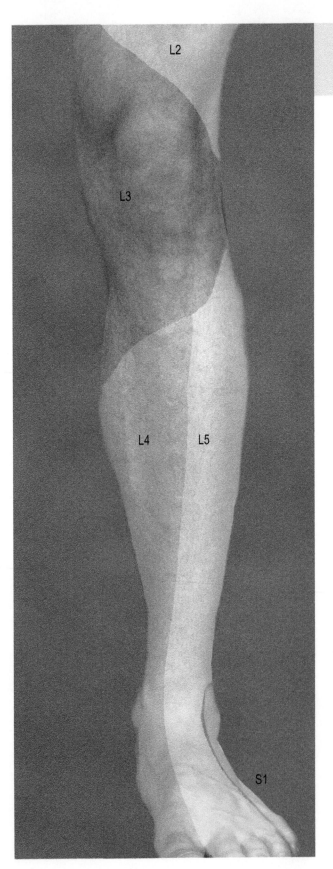

Figure A.8

Lower limb dermatomes

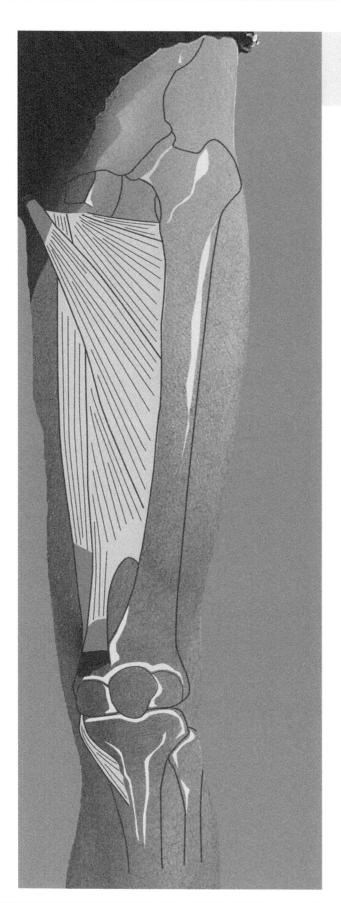

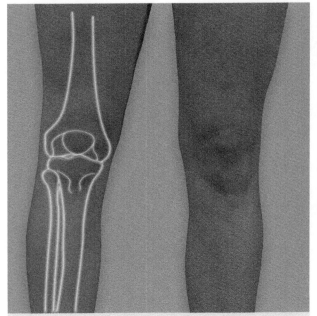

Figure A.10

Bony landmarks, right knee

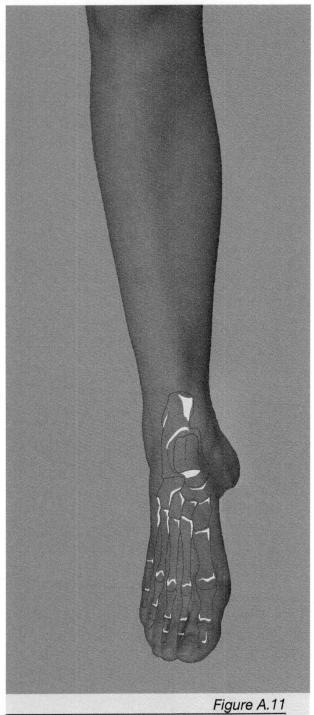

Figure A.11

Bones of the foot

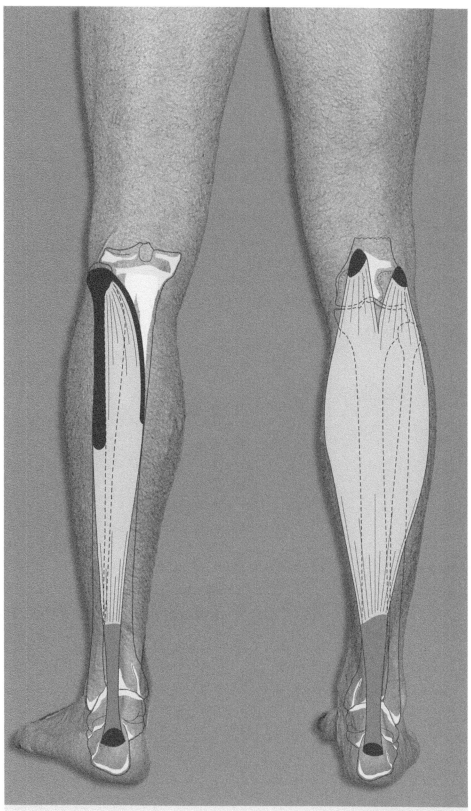

Figure A.12

Soleus (left side)   **Gastrocnemius (right side)**

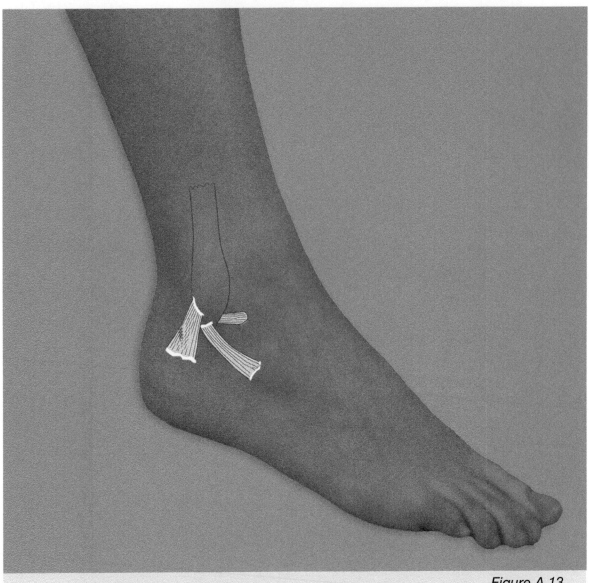

Figure A.13

Lateral ligaments at the ankle

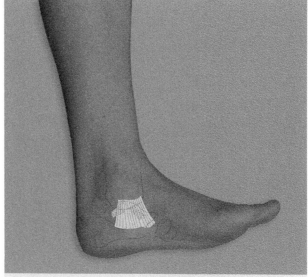

Figure A.15

Deltoid ligament at the ankle

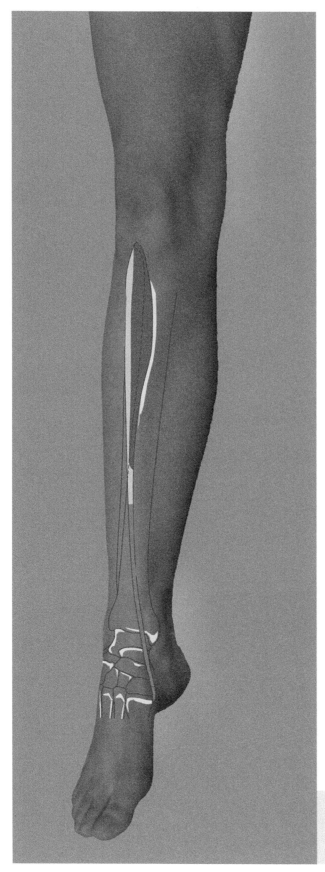

Figure A.14

Tibialis anterior

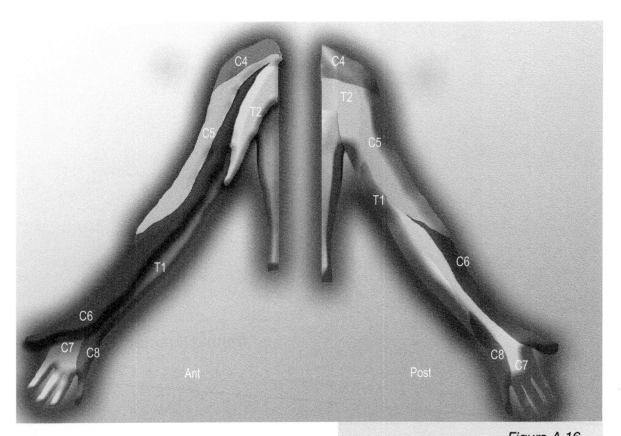

Figure A.16

Dermatomes of the arm

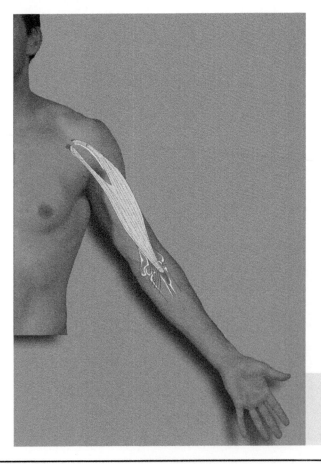

Figure A.17

Biceps

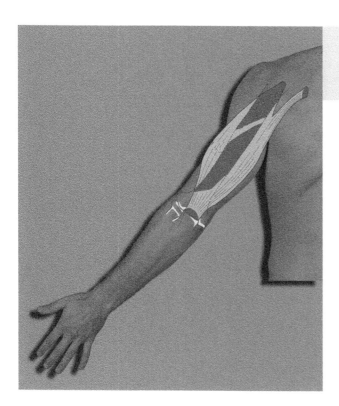

Figure A.18

Triceps brachii

Figure A.19

Surface anatomy upper limb

lateral end of clavicle	1
acromioclavicular joint	2
deltoid	3
biceps brachii	4
triceps	5
pectoralis major sternal fibres	6
pectoralis major clavicular fibres	7
common extensor origin	8
common flexor origin	9
flexor muscles of the forearm	10
wrist joint	11
thenar eminence	12
hypothenar eminence	13

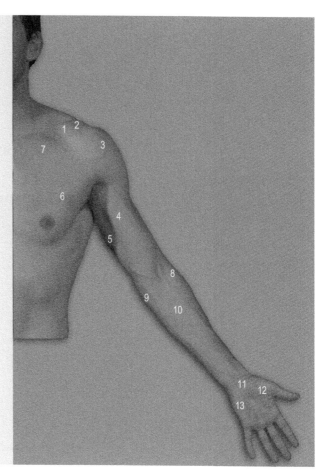

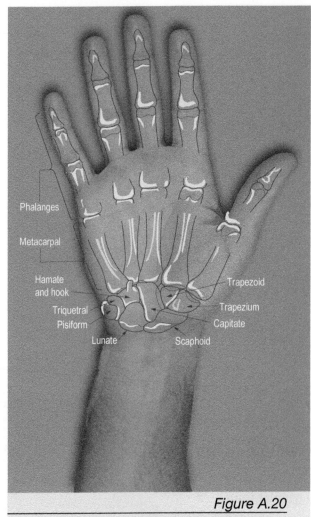

Phalanges

Metacarpal

Hamate
and hook

Triquetral

Pisiform

Lunate

Trapezoid

Trapezium

Capitate

Scaphoid

Figure A.20

Bones of the hand

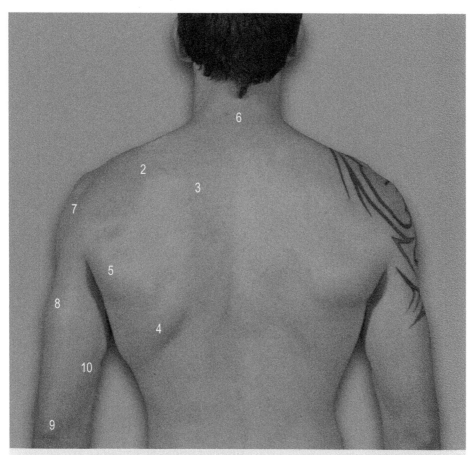

Figure A.21

Surface marking of the posterior shoulder and thorax

supraspinatus	2
medial border of scapula	3
inferior angle of scapula	4
teres major	5
C7 spinous process	6
deltoid	7
lateral head of triceps	8
olecranon process	9
medial head of triceps	10

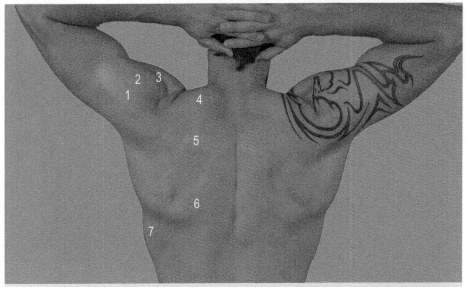

Figure A.22

Muscles of the posterior shoulder and thorax

posterior fibres deltoid	1
middle fibres deltoid	2
anterior fibres deltoid	3
upper fibres trapezius	4
rhomboids	5
inferior angle of scapula	6
latissimus dorsi	7

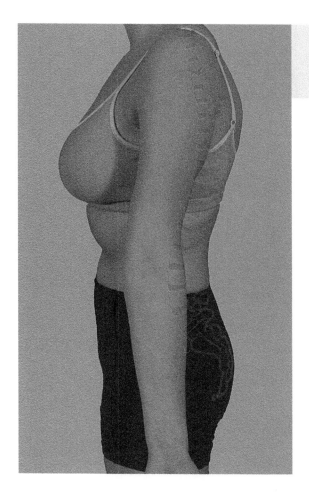

Figure A.23

The curves of the spine

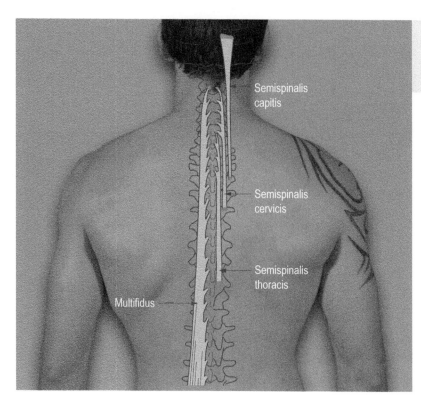

Figure A.24

Erector spinae

Semispinalis
capitis

Semispinalis
cervicis

Semispinalis
thoracis

Multifidus

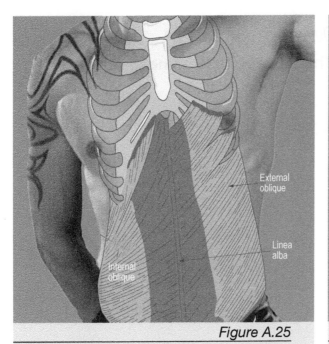

Figure A.25

Internal and external oblique muscles

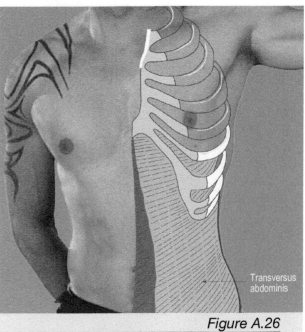

Figure A.26

Transversus abdominis

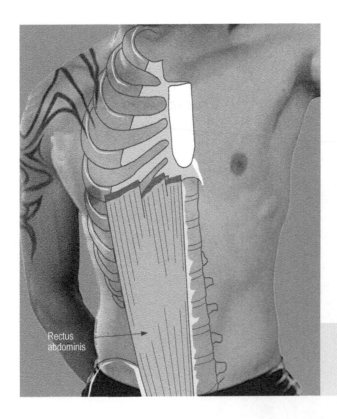

Figure A.27

Rectus abdominis

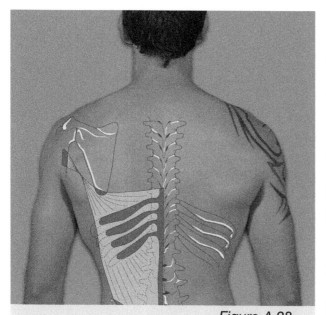

Figure A.28

Latissimus dorsi

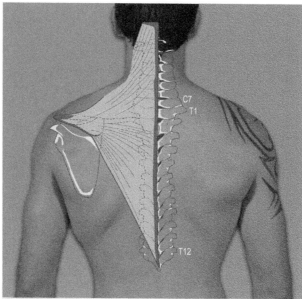

Figure A.29

Supraspinatus

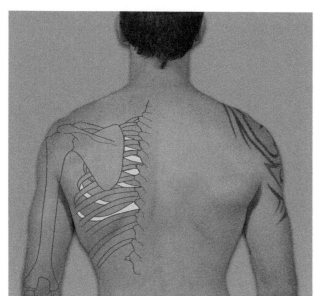

Figure A.30

Bony landmarks of the posterior arm and thorax

Figure A.31

Trapezius

Figure A.32

Pelvis and femur, anterior view

iliac crest	1
anterior superior iliac spine	2
anterior inferior iliac spine	3
head of femur	4
neck of femur	5
greater trochanter	6
intertrochanteric line	7
lesser trochanter	8
shaft of femur	9
pubic symphysis	10
ischial tuberosity	11
ischial spine	12
iliac surface of sacroiliac joint	13
ilium	14
posterior superior iliac spine	15
posterior inferior iliac spine	16

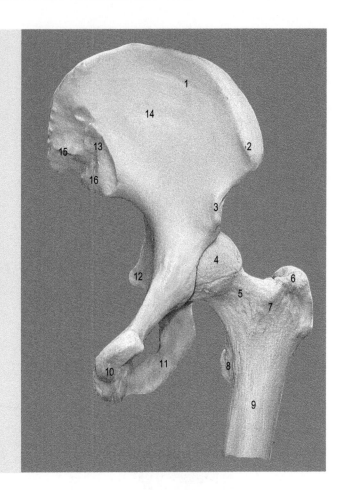

Figure A.33

Lateral view of pelvis

anterior superior iliac spine	1
anterior inferior iliac spine	2
iliac crest	3
posterior superior iliac spine	4
posterior inferior iliac spine	5
position of acetabular labrum	6
acetabulum	7
ischial tuberosity	8
pubis	9
position of obturator membrane in obturator foramen	10

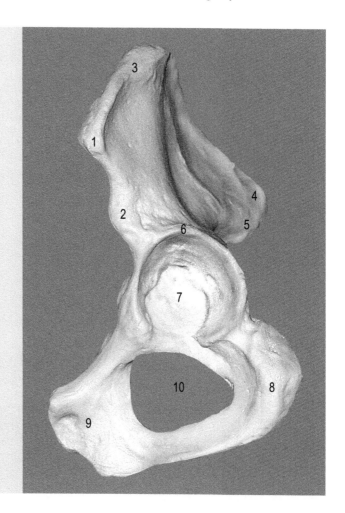

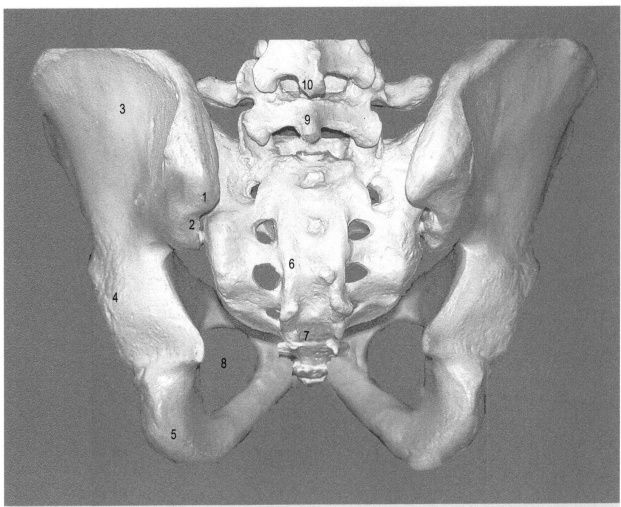

Figure A.34

Posterior of pelvis

posterior superior iliac spine	1
posterior inferior iliac spine	2
ilium	3
acetabulum	4
ischial tuberosity	5
sacrum	6
coccyx	7
obturator foramen	8
5th lumbar vertebra	9
4th lumbar vertebra	10

Figure A.35

Proximal femur

greater trochanter	1
lesser trochanter	2
intertrochanteric line (crest at posterior)	3
neck of femur	4
head of femur	5
shaft of femur	6

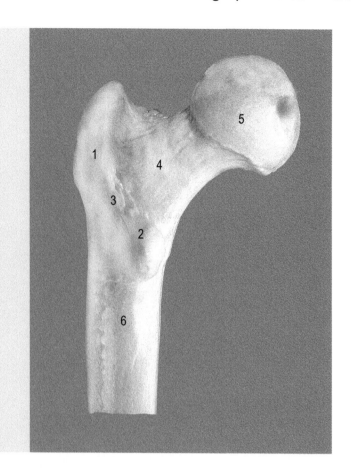

Figure A.36

The knee joint

shaft of femur	1
lateral femoral epicondyle	2
lateral femoral condyle	3
medial femoral condyle	4
adductor tubercle	5
medial tibial condyle	6
lateral tibial condyle	7
tibial tuberosity	8
superior tibiofibular joint	9
head of fibula	10

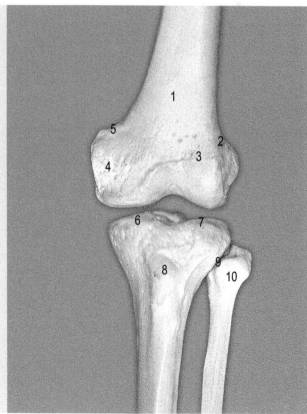

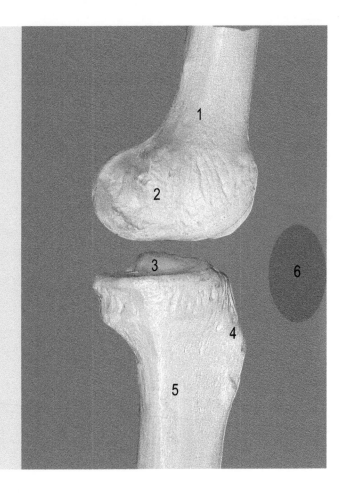

Figure A.37

Knee joint, medial view

shaft of femur	1
medial condyle	2
tibial spine	3
tibial tuberosity	4
shaft of tibia	5
position of patella	6

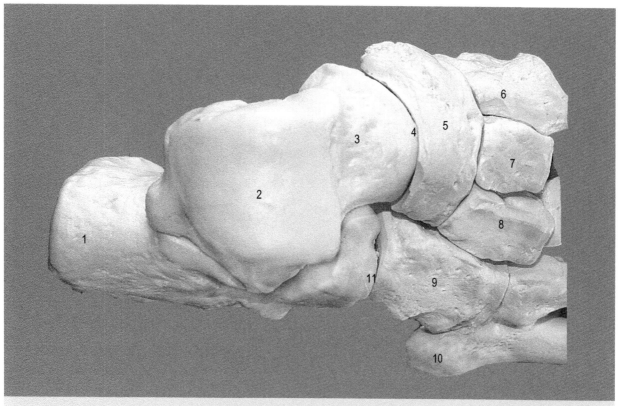

Figure A.38

Right foot, superior aspect

calcaneus	1
superior aspect of talus that forms ankle joint	2
head of talus	3
talocalcaneonavicular joint	4
navicular	5
cuneiforms	6,7,8
cuboid	9
tubercle at base of 5th metatarsal	10
calcaneocuboid joint	11

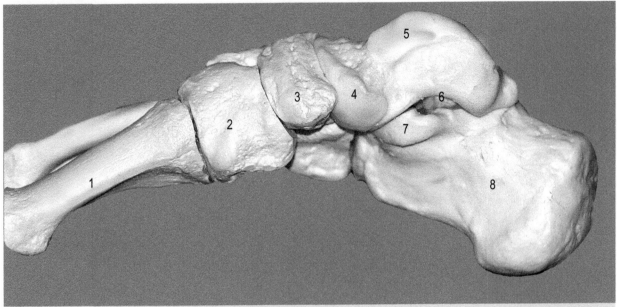

Figure A.39

Right foot, medial aspect

1st metatarsal	1
medial cuneiform	2
navicular	3
head of talus	4
talus	5
subtalar joint	6
sustentaculum tali	7
calcaneus	8

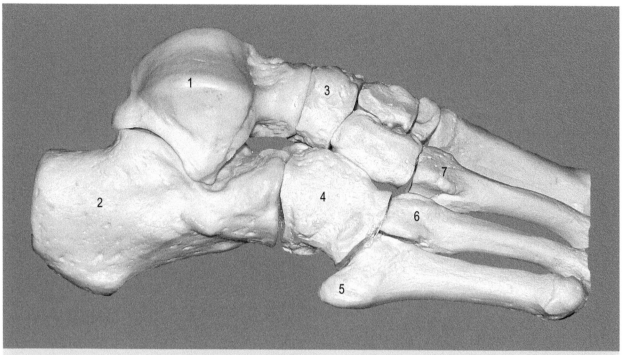

Figure A.40

Right foot, lateral aspect

talus	1
calcaneus	2
navicular	3
cuboid	4
tubercle at base of 5th metatarsal	5
4th metatarsal	6
3rd metatarsal	7

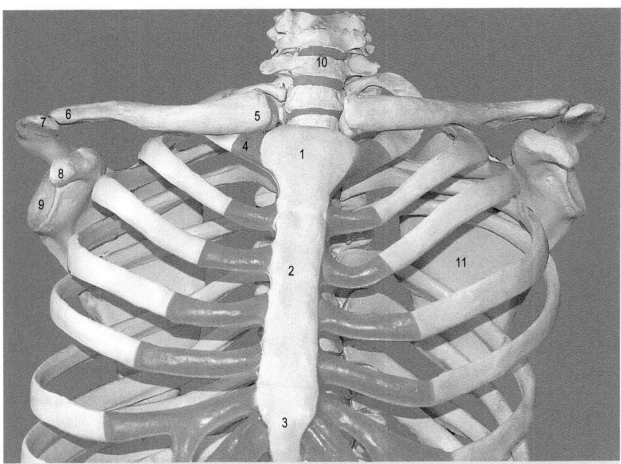

Figure A.41

Thorax, from front

manubrium	1
sternum	2
xiphoid process	3
first rib	4
medial end of clavicle ending in sternoclavicular joint	5
lateral end of clavicle ending in acromioclavicular joint	6
acromion process	7
coracoid process	8
glenoid fossa	9
cervical vertebrae	10
anterior surface of scapula sitting on chest wall	11

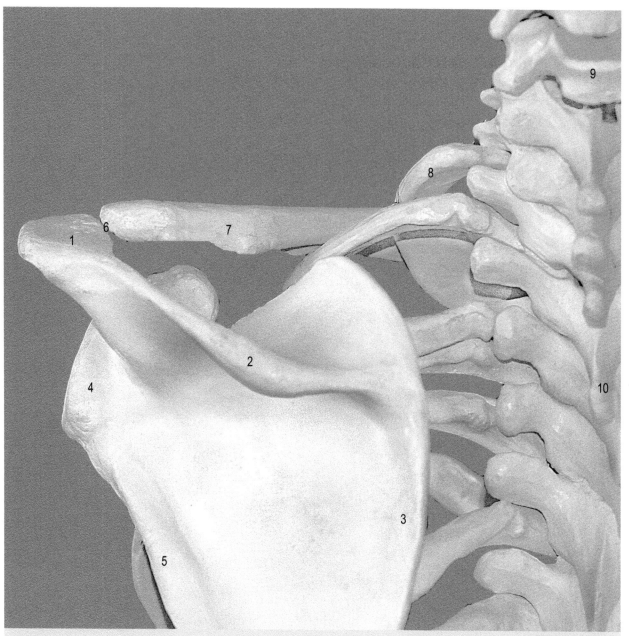

Figure A.42

Posterior thorax including left scapula

1	acromion process	acromioclavicular joint	6
2	spine of scapula	clavicle	7
3	medial end of scapula	first rib	8
4	glenoid	cervical spine	9
5	lateral border of scapula	thoracic spine	10

Figure A.43

Right elbow, posterior view

medial epicondyle	1
olecranon	2
lateral epicondyle	3
shaft of ulna	4
head of radius	5
shaft of radius	6

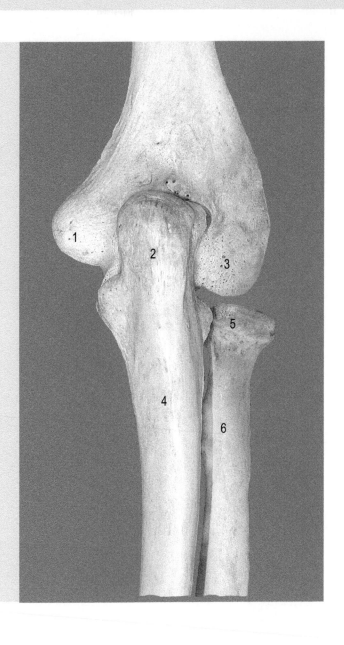

Figure A.44

Right elbow, anterior view

shaft of humerus	1
lateral supracondylar ridge	2
medial supracondylar ridge	3
capitulum	4
trochlea	5
head of radius	6
coronoid process	7
radial tuberosity	8
shaft of radius	9
shaft of ulna	10

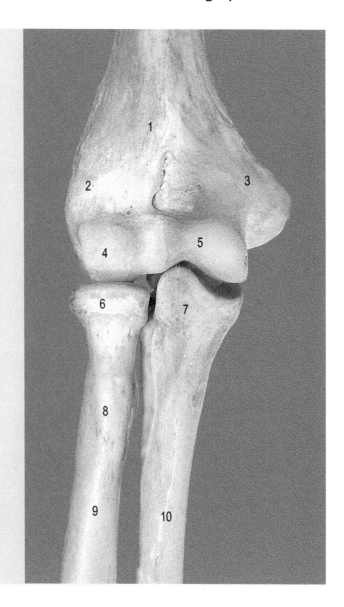

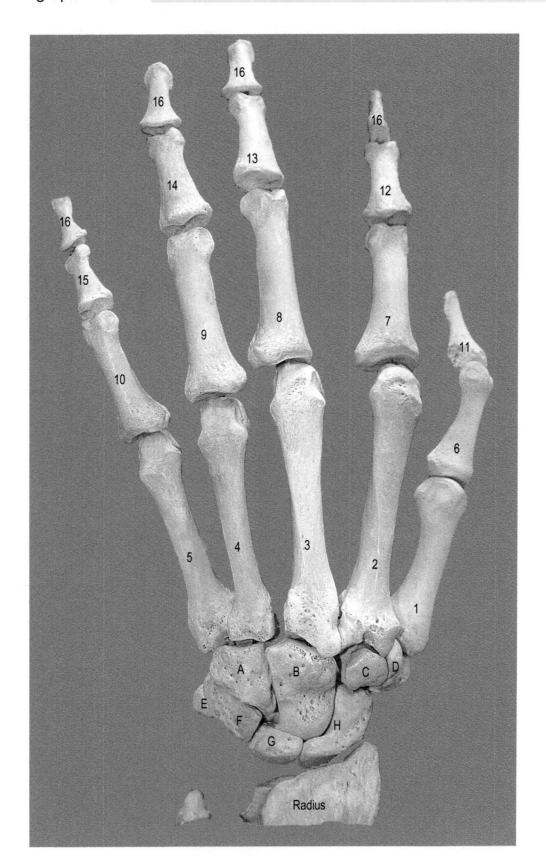

Figure A.45
_____

Left hand, dorsal view

1	first metacarpal
2	second metacarpal
3	third metacarpal
4	fourth metacarpal
5	fifth metacarpal
6	first proximal phalanx
7	second proximal phalanx
8	third proximal phalanx
9	fourth proximal phalanx
10	fifth proximal phalanx
11	distal phalanx
12,13,14,15	intermediate phalanges
16	distal phalanges

carpal bones

A hamate

B capitate

C trapezoid

D trapezium

E pisiform

F triquetral

G lunate

H scaphoid

Figure A.46

Right humerus, anterior view

humeral head	1
lesser tubercle	2
intertubercular sulcus (biceps tendon goes through here)	3
greater tubercle	4
shaft	5

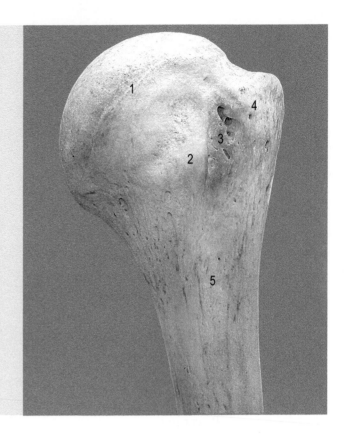

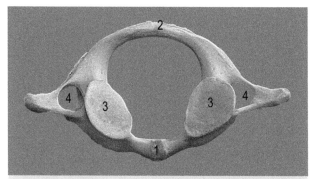

Figure A.47

C1 from above

anterior arch	1
posterior arch	2
articular facet	3
foramen transversarium	4

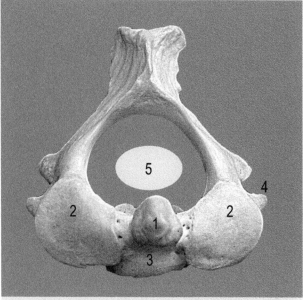

Figure A.48

C2 from above

odontoid	1
articular facet	2
vertebral body	3
transverse process	4
neural canal	5

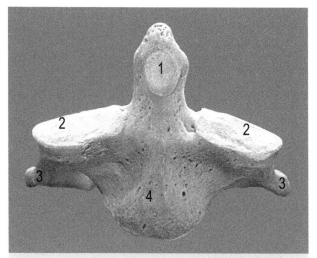

Figure A.49

C2 from front

odontoid	1
articular facet	2
transverse process	3
vertebral body	4

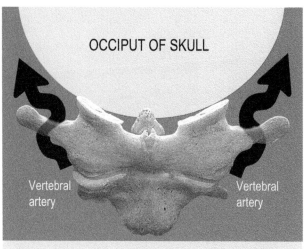

OCCIPUT OF SKULL

Vertebral artery

Vertebral artery

Figure A.50

C1 and C2 articulated together

note the path of the vertebral artery

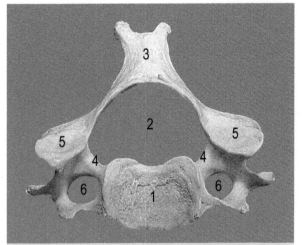

Figure A.51

A typical cervical vertebra

vertebral body (small)	1
neural canal (large)	2
spinous process (bifid, or forked)	3
transverse process	4
articular facet	5
foramen transversarium (vertebral artery goes through here)	6

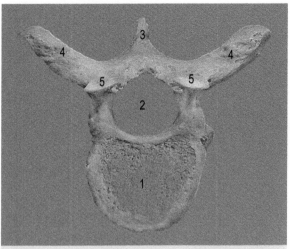

Figure A.52

Typical thoracic vertebra

vertebral body	1
neural canal (triangular)	2
spinous process (angled downwards)	3
transverse process	4
facet joint (aligned to allow rotation)	5

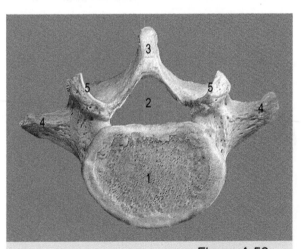

Figure A.53

Typical lumbar vertebra

vertebral body	1
neural canal	2
spinous process	3
transverse process	4
facet joint (aligned to block rotation)	5

Bibliography

Aagaard, H. and Verdonk, R. (1999). Function of the normal meniscus and consequences of meniscal resection. *Scand J Med Sci Sports* **9**(3): 134–40.

Adams, M. A., Freeman, B. J. *et al.* (2000). Mechanical initiation of intervertebral disc degeneration. *Spine* **25**(13): 1625–36.

Ahmad, I. (1975). Articular muscle of the knee – articularis genus. *Bull Hosp Joint Dis* **36**(1): 58–60.

Andrews, J. R., Carson, W. G., Jr. *et al.* (1985). Glenoid labrum tears related to the long head of the biceps. *Am J Sports Med* **13**(5): 337–41.

Bagg, S. D. and Forrest, W. J. (1988). A biomechanical analysis of scapular rotation during arm abduction in the scapular plane. *Am J Phys Med Rehabil* **67**(6): 238–45.

Bogduk, N., Johnson, G. *et al.* (1998). The morphology and biomechanics of latissimus dorsi. *Clin Biomech (Bristol, Avon)* **13**(6): 377–85.

Cober, S. R. and Trumble, T. E. (2001). Arthroscopic repair of triangular fibrocartilage complex injuries. *Orthop Clin North Am* **32**(2): 279–94, viii.

Dolan, P. and Adams, M. A. (1998). Repetitive lifting tasks fatigue the back muscles and increase the bending moment acting on the lumbar spine. *J Biomech* **31**(8): 713–21.

Englund, M., Roos, E. M. *et al.* (2001). Patient-relevant outcomes fourteen years after meniscectomy: influence of type of meniscal tear and size of resection. *Rheumatology (Oxford)* **40**(6): 631–9.

Fischer-Rasmussen, T. and Jensen, P. E. (2000). Proprioceptive sensitivity and performance in anterior cruciate ligament-deficient knee joints. *Scand J Med Sci Sports* **10**(2): 85–9.

Giddings, V. L., Beaupre, G. S. *et al.* (2000). Calcaneal loading during walking and running. *Med Sci Sports Exerc* **32**(3): 627–34.

Goto, H., Shuler, F. D. *et al.* (2000). Gene therapy for meniscal injury: enhanced synthesis of proteoglycan and collagen by meniscal cells transduced with a TGFbeta(1)gene. *Osteoarthritis Cartilage* **8**(4): 266–71.

Guiot, B. H. and Fessler, R. G. (2000). Molecular biology of degenerative disc disease. *Neurosurgery* **47**(5): 1034–40.

Hunt, A. E., Smith, R. M. *et al.* (2001). Extrinsic muscle activity, foot motion and ankle joint moments during the stance phase of walking. *Foot Ankle Int* **22**(1): 31–41.

Jobe, C. M. (1996). Superior glenoid impingement. Current concepts. *Clin Orthop* **330**: 98–107.

Kido, T., Itoi, E. *et al.* (2000). The depressor function of biceps on the head of the humerus in shoulders with tears of the rotator cuff. *J Bone Joint Surg Br* **82**(3): 416–19.

Makris, C. A., Georgoulis, A. D. *et al.* (2000). Posterior cruciate ligament architecture: evaluation under microsurgical dissection. *Arthroscopy* **16**(6): 627–32.

Michiels, I. and Grevenstein, J. (1995). Kinematics of shoulder abduction in the scapular plane. On the influence of abduction velocity and external load. *Clin Biomech (Bristol, Avon)* **10**(3): 137–43.

Nadler, S. F., Malanga, G. A. *et al.* (2001). Relationship between hip muscle imbalance and occurrence of low back pain in collegiate athletes: a prospective study. *Am J Phys Med Rehabil* **80**(8): 572–7.

Rodeo, S. A. (2001). Meniscal allografts – where do we stand? *Am J Sports Med* **29**(2): 246–61.

Sanan, A. and Rengachary, S. S. (1996). The history of spinal biomechanics. *Neurosurgery* **39**(4): 657–68; discussion 668–9.

Santaguida, P. L. and McGill, S. M. (1995). The psoas major muscle: a three-dimensional geometric study. *J Biomech* **28**(3): 339–45.

Self, B. P., Harris, S. *et al.* (2000). Ankle biomechanics during impact landings on uneven surfaces. *Foot Ankle Int* **21**(2): 138–44.

Simunic, D. I., Broom, N. D. *et al.* (2001). Biomechanical factors influencing nuclear disruption of the intervertebral disc. *Spine* **26**(11): 1223–30.

Swanepoel, M. W., Adams, L. M. *et al.* (1995). Human lumbar apophyseal joint damage and intervertebral disc degeneration. *Ann Rheum Dis* **54**(3): 182–8.

Thompson, R. E., Pearcy, M. J. *et al.* (2000). Disc lesions and the mechanics of the intervertebral joint complex. *Spine* **25**(23): 3026–35.

Wang, M. and Dumas, G. A. (1998). Mechanical behavior of the female sacroiliac joint and influence of the anterior and posterior sacroiliac ligaments under sagittal loads. *Clin Biomech (Bristol, Avon)* **13**(4–5): 293–9.

Yoshizawa, H., O'Brien, J. P. *et al.* (1980). The neuropathology of intervertebral discs removed for low-back pain. *J Pathol* **132**(2): 95–104.

Index

Printed and bound by CPI Group (UK) Ltd, Croydon, CR0 4YY

03/10/2024

01040345-0020